Forever Young

A Journey into Anti-Aging and Longevity

by
Steven Walker

Table of Contents

Introduction:
Embracing the Ageless Journey

Time, with its steady drumbeat, marches on, slipping through our fingers like the grains of sand in an hourglass. Yet, as we trace the arc of human history and our unrelenting quest for vitality, it becomes abundantly clear that the pursuit of a life well lived is as timeless as the stars. The emphasis on longevity — a dance with time that seeks not merely the extension of years, but the enrichment of life within those years — illuminates every culture's narrative, carving out stories of elixirs, fables of fountains of youth, and myriad quests for the secret of perpetual vitality.

Now, equipped with an arsenal of burgeoning scientific knowledge, a resolute spirit, and the universal desire to harness the proverbial fountain, we find ourselves at the precipice of a new era in human health. In this handbook of sorts, we embark on a journey that's not about running away from aging, but rather embracing it with grace, understanding, and proactive zeal.

Aging, after all, isn't merely the byproduct of time's passage; it's a sophisticated biological process influenced by a confluence of factors. Genetics, lifestyle choices, the environment, and even our emotional state interlace to sculpt the story of our advancing years. And embedded within this intricate web is a profound truth: a lifestyle that acknowledges and adapts to these myriad elements can profoundly enhance one's well-being, vitality, and the length of an optimally lived life.

Consider this introduction a gateway, an opening passage that beckons with promise and empowerment. We're setting the stage for a transformative exploration, one that doesn't shy away from the science of aging but rather makes it an ally. The marvels of our biological clock, the fascinating interplay with our genetic tapestry, are just the beginning of what's to come.

The mind, a universe within itself, holds pivotal sway over our perception of aging. It's not just the physiological but the psychological facets of aging we'll navigate, understanding how our mental framing can have tangible effects on our longevity. For isn't it said that the body listens to the mind's whispers and sometimes even its silent musings?

Nutrition, a cornerstone of good health, also takes center stage. We'll delve into the very building blocks of life — essential nutrients, nature's bounty of superfoods, and the dietary practices echoing through time and culture that contribute to a life protracted and enriched.

The elixir of life isn't a mythical concoction but flows abundantly from our taps. Hydration and its undeniable connection with aging receives its fair share of the spotlight, highlighting that the quality of the lifeblood that circulates within us is quintessential to the journey of aging gracefully.

As our expedition into longevity unfolds, so does our understanding of the body's need for movement. Like a symphony, it requires a conductor — the right exercises and personal fitness plans that are akin to a fine-tuned arrangement promoting endurance, strength, and the elegance of mobility.

And what of rest — the sweet repose that rejuvenates and restores? Explore how the gentle embrace of slumber can be a fountain of youth in its own right — the rightful periods of rest an antidote to the wear and tear of days well seized.

Stress, with its aging acceleration, is a dragon that we all must learn to tame. Herein, we'll equip ourselves with the shield and sword of stress management techniques that rebuff the advances of time's withering effects.

The canvas of our skin tells a story — one that need not be of decline but of preservation and reverence. We shall uncover the secrets to skin care that honor the vessel we inhabit.

Our internal cascade of hormones, endlessly ebbing and flowing, wields significant power in our aging narrative. Understanding and maintaining this delicate balance is akin to orchestrating an internal harmony that resounds through the years.

And let us not forget the quintessence of our essence — the brain. Cognitive function, mental acuity, and brain health lay the foundation for an ageless mind within its neurological bastion.

We live not in isolation, but in the rich tapestry of human connection. The pulsating strength of our social ties has a potent and palpable impact on our longevity. As we unveil the robust threads that bind us, we understand just how interwoven our wellbeing and our world truly are.

From the roots of ancient botanical wisdom emerge the modern insights of supplemental science. Like a discerning gardener, we shall learn which vitamins, minerals, and herbal comforts may be lovingly added to the soil of our wellbeing to flourish with the passing seasons.

As each chapter unfurls, the ageless journey will beckon us through meandering paths — alternative therapies, detoxification for rejuvenation, avant-garde medical advancements, and personalized medicine will all offer us glimpses into the wellspring of youth.

We stand, all of us, on the threshold of an ageless journey. A journey not confined to the fleetingness of youth but expanding into the embrace of a life deeply and richly experienced. This is an invitation — one that extends to health-conscious individuals everywhere. An invitation to embrace, navigate, and cherish every turning of the day and night as part of a grander, more resplendent journey.

So let's begin, not with trepidation but with the vigor of explorers charting a course through the waters of time. Let us engage with the intricate beauty of aging, not as an inevitable descent but as an ascent to wisdom, wellness, and a life's worth of moments cherished and embraced. For indeed, the future can be forever young to those who prepare and proceed with enlightened knowledge, compassionate self-care, and an unwavering commitment to the art of living fully at every age.

Chapter 1:
The Science of Aging

A s we turn the page from our introduction, the complexities of aging beckon us into a fascinating territory where science, like a skilled artist, paints the many shades of our biological journey. The pursuit of longevity isn't merely about adding years to life, but infusing those years with vitality, and the keystone to that pursuit rests within the intricate workings of our body's biological clock. Understanding the mechanisms that tick away with precision isn't an esoteric pursuit – it's our gateway to harnessing control over how we age. While genetics toss us the dice with a smirk, hinting at predetermined fates, the reality couldn't be more interactive. Our genes don't dictate; they converse with our choices, our environment, and our attitudes toward life itself. This chapter delves into the heart of aging, dissecting the role that genetics play in our personal longevity narrative and uncovering the myriad ways we can influence the ticking of our own biological clocks. It's a tale of intertwined destinies, a story that explores not only the 'how' but also the 'why' behind the waltz of our cells and molecules as we glide through the passage of time.

Understanding the Biological Clock As we delve into the intricacies of our biological clock, it's essential to understand that this isn't some abstract concept. It's a tangible, physiological process that ticks away deep within our cells, orchestrating the symphony of hormones, cellular repair, and regeneration that dictates our pace of aging. It's the metronome to which our bodily functions harmonize, guiding everything from sleep cycles to our metabolism.

The term 'circadian rhythm' often pops up when discussing the biological clock. It refers to the roughly 24-hour cycle in the physiological processes of living beings. Not just a human thing, mind you; plants, animals, and even tiny microbes experience these daily rhythms. These rhythms are influenced by external cues like light and darkness and dictate when we feel alert or sleepy, among other processes.

But let's dig a notch deeper. The master clock controlling these rhythms lies in a part of your brain called the suprachiasmatic nucleus (SCN), a group of cells in the hypothalamus. This cluster of neurons takes cues from the environment, particularly light, and sends signals throughout the body to regulate temperature, release hormones, and manage energy levels, all in a day's work.

Melatonin, the 'sleep hormone,' serves as a night-time messenger. At dusk, as the light dims, the SCN nudges the pineal gland to secrete melatonin, signaling that it's time to wind down. Come morning, light shuts this process down, cueing a wake-up call for the body. It's an intricate dance between our internal physiology and the external world's rhythms.

However, it's not just about sleep. The biological clock affects our digestion, heart rate, and even how our body metabolizes medications. Disturbances in our circadian rhythm, such as those caused by shift work or jet lag, can lead to a variety of health problems, echoing the age-old advice that routine is key to good health.

What's fascinating is that almost every cell in your body has its own mini-clock. These peripheral clocks ensure that various processes are optimized for certain times of the day. They are responsible for when certain genes are turned on and off or when cells divide and repair themselves—critical functions for maintaining youthfulness and staving off the tell-tale signs of aging.

As we age, our biological clock's accuracy can falter. It gets a bit wonky, and the once precise signaling can become more akin to static on a radio. The outcome? Desynchronized bodily functions can lead to sleep disorders, weight problems, and even an increased risk for chronic conditions like heart disease and diabetes.

Emerging research indicates that lifestyle factors can also influence the integrity of our biological clock. Everything from exposure to artificial light at night, irregular meal times, to lack of physical activity, can play a role. It suggests that aligning our habits with our natural circadian rhythms could be instrumental in anti-aging efforts.

Interestingly, some studies suggest that fasting and caloric restriction can strengthen the biological clock's functioning. By creating a clear feeding-fasting cycle, you might help reset and reinforce those clocks in your cells, potentially slowing down some aspects of aging.

It's also worth pointing out that chronotype — whether you're a morning lark or a night owl — is influenced by genetic elements of our biological clock. Those natural preferences for waking and sleeping times are built into our DNA, and going against them can create internal chaos. Respecting your unique chronotype can be critical for optimizing health and longevity.

Moreover, the strength and consistency of the daily light-dark cycle we're exposed to can enhance or impair our biological clock's performance. Modern life has a way of blurring the lines between day and night, but sticking to routines that respect natural light patterns can synchronize our internal clocks for the better.

Even the microbiome — the community of microorganisms living in our digestive tract — operates on a circadian rhythm. These tiny inhabitants play a role in digestion, immunity, and even mood, and their well-being is interlaced with our own through the language of the biological clock.

And let's not forget, as we whisper the importance of sleep, that this isn't merely about quantity. The quality of sleep matters deeply, too. Sleep phases need to move with the grace of a well-rehearsed quartet, and disruptions in this progression can have cascading effects on how, and how well, we age.

Ultimately, the biological clock runs the show in how we move through the days and years. Respecting this clock, keeping it well-oiled and synchronized, appears to be central to the pursuit of longevity. Our task, then, is to live in harmony with this internal timepiece, gracefully setting the pace for a vibrant life today, tomorrow, and well into the future.

In conclusion, the biological clock is a complex but exceedingly elegant system comprising cellular and hormonal rhythms. As more research unfolds, the adage to "listen to your body" takes on new, profound meaning. By understanding and living in tune with the natural cadence set by our biological clock, we edge closer to that fountain of youthful living, one timely tick at a time.

The Role of Genetics in Longevity Now, as we delve deeper into the connection between our genetic makeup and the aging process, it's imperative to understand that the human body is akin to an incredibly intricate orchestra. Each gene represents a musician, contributing their unique sound to the collective symphony of life. Indeed, our genetics play a dynamic role in determining not just how we age, but also our potential lifespan.

Let's first establish that longevity is not merely a result of one or two "fountain of youth" genes. Instead, it's a complex interaction among a multitude of genes, each influencing various pathways that drive the aging process. Several studies, including those centered on family history and twins, suggest a substantial genetic component to long life. If your parents and grandparents waved a cheerful goodbye to their 90s before departing this world, there's a fair chance that you could follow in their centenarian footsteps, at least in part due to your inherited DNA.

One can't talk genetics without mentioning the role of telomeres, the protective caps at the ends of our chromosomes. Like the plastic tips on shoelaces, telomeres prevent chromosomes from fraying, which would otherwise lead to a loss of important genetic information. As we age, our telomeres shorten, and telomere length has been linked to lifespan. Scientists have found individuals with longer telomeres tend to live longer, healthier lives. This begs the question: could we slow aging by preserving telomere length?

Genome-wide association studies (GWAS) have identified certain genes that are more prevalent in individuals who live to an old age. Among these is the well-studied APOE gene, which comes in several variants. One of these, APOE e4, is associated with an increased risk of Alzheimer's disease, while APOE e2 is linked to a longer lifespan. The FOXO gene family, particularly FOXO3, also emerges frequently in conversations about longevity, thanks to its role in repairing DNA and regulating oxidative stress.

Interestingly, the genetic predisposition for a longer life doesn't come without its caveats. For instance, longevity genes may also prepare the body well for combating stress, disease, and dietary excesses. In other words, people who live exceptionally long lives may not only have 'good genes' but also genes that respond robustly to life's challenges.

Nevertheless, genes are only part of the story. They certainly set the stage, but the environment and lifestyle choices crank the spotlight and cue the music. Someone may have genetics that favor longevity, but without a healthy environment and good life habits, their genetic advantage might not be fully realized. The theory of genetic penetrance comes into play here; just because you have a gene doesn't mean its traits will express completely or at all, depending on external factors.

Evidence also shows that behaviors and environmental influences can affect our genetic expression through a process called epigenetics, where chemical modifications can turn genes on or off without changing the DNA sequence itself. As such, someone can optimize their genetic potential for a longer life by aligning their lifestyle with what's considered beneficial for healthy aging—managing stress, eating a balanced diet, staying physically active, and avoiding harmful substances and environments.

For those intrigued by the potential of manipulating genetics to extend life, current science is exploring gene editing. CRISPR technology, for instance, allows scientists to make precise edits to the DNA, raising the possibility of one day being able to correct mutations that contribute to early aging or diseases linked to aging. While still in its infancy regarding clinical applications for longevity, gene editing opens a box of ethical questions along with its potential.

Now, don't fall into the trap of thinking genetics is destiny. Yes, the genetic lottery hands out tickets at birth, but the numbers on these tickets can change throughout our lifetime. Lifestyle can be seen as a wildcard, altering the outcome of the lottery by promoting genetic expressions that are beneficial to longevity.

A look into the burgeoning field of nutrigenomics shows the dance between genes and diet. This discipline suggests that personalized nutrition based on an individual's genetic makeup can be pivotal for longevity. By understanding genetic variants and how they respond to different nutrients, one could tailor a diet that reduces disease risk and promotes a longer life.

Moving beyond nutrition, even our social surroundings can help shape our epigenetic profiles. Positive social interactions and a supportive community have been associated with beneficial epigenetic changes, a reflection of the profound impact of our social environment on our biology.

When pondering the future of aging, it's clear that genetics will remain a key player. Advancements in understanding our genome and how it interacts with the myriad aspects of our lives will lead to more informed decisions regarding health and longevity. While the promise of personalized genetic intervention is on the horizon, the realization of a life fully optimized for longevity will likely depend on a symphony of lifestyle harmonization.

The scientific journey into the role of genetics in longevity is an ongoing voyage of discovery. For those of us aiming to live a long and flourishing life, this knowledge empowers us to navigate the aging process with a sense of control and optimism. Our genetics offer a map, but ultimately, we are the captains charting the course of our own health journey, adjusting the sails as we respond to the winds of lifestyle, environment, and personal choices.

Take heart in the fact that we're learning more every day. Each study and every scientific endeavor brings us closer to understanding just how powerful our genes can be when supported by the pillars of a healthy lifestyle. While we may not have control over the genes we inherit, the understanding of their influence on longevity is a golden key to unlocking the potential for a well-lived, vibrant existence as we age. It's a beautiful harmony of nature and nurture, dancing through the timeline of our lives.

Chapter 2:
The Psychology of Aging

As we transition from the fascinating realm of our biological clocks and genetic influences on longevity, we pivot to focus on the mental and emotional frameworks that underpin our experience of growing older. The psychology of aging isn't just about the passage of time but about the narratives we weave around each year that passes. We'll explore how our perception of aging affects not just the way we feel about those silver strands in our hair but can also tangibly influence our physical health and lifespan. With an understanding that a youthful mindset isn't just a platitude but a powerful tool, we'll dive into cognitive strategies that can keep our spirits dancing even when our joints aren't as enthusiastic. Embracing the psychological facets of aging allows us to retain a sense of control and joy as the pages of the calendar turn, ensuring that we don't just add years to our lives, but life to our years.

Perception of Age and Its Impact on Longevity If you've ever been told you're only as old as you feel, there might be more truth to that statement than you'd think. The way we perceive our age and the aging process has profound implications for our longevity. What's fascinating is that our mind's eye can exert a powerful influence on the body's biological clock. This place where psychology dovetails with biology is where some of the most exciting—and underappreciated—anti-aging strategies lie.

Consider how the perception of age influences behavior. When people view age as a barrier, they're less likely to engage in physical activity or seek new experiences, leading to a more sedentary lifestyle. In contrast, those who perceive aging as a series of opportunities tend to maintain a more active, engaged lifestyle. This difference in outlook isn't just about morale; it's about how our cells and systems function.

Let's take a closer look at the power of mindset. Research suggests that individuals with a positive self-perception of aging live longer than those with a negative one. It's not magic—it's mindset. By fostering a more positive view of aging, we can potentially unlock inner reserves of resilience and vitality.

Our belief systems about aging are shaped early and continue to evolve throughout life. It's not just society's narrative about aging that matters, but the stories we tell ourselves. If we can shift these internal narratives from decline to growth, we signal to our brain that we're still in the game, still growing, still developing—still living.

It's not just about longevity for the sake of additional years. The quality of those years is paramount. Studies have shown that a youthful outlook can result in better health outcomes, including reduced risk of chronic disease, better mental health, and improved cognitive function. This is the rich, intertwined tapestry of belief influencing biology.

But how does one begin to foster a more youthful perception of age? Start by challenging ingrained stereotypes you might hold about aging. There's a compelling case for auditing the media we consume and the language we use when talking about age. After all, if we constantly bombard ourselves with messages that equate aging with decline, we're wiring our brains to accept this as an inevitable truth.

Cultivating an environment that supports a youthful outlook is also critical. From the company we keep to the passions we pursue, everything sends a signal back to our psyche about our place in life's timeline. Engaging with diverse age groups and pursuing lifelong learning can reinforce a sense of ongoing growth and vitality.

The physical dimension of this outlook is just as vital. While we'll address specific exercises in later chapters, it's worth noting here that regular physical activity is a vessel for a youthful mindset. It enhances vitality and energy levels, which in turn reinforces a positive self-perception of age. Remember, the body and mind are in constant conversation, and exercise is one of their most fluent languages.

Don't underestimate the ritual of self-care and its psychological benefits either. When we take care of our appearance, engage in skin-care routines, or dress in ways that make us feel confident, we send a powerful message to the brain: we matter, we are valued, and we are not defined by the number of years we've been around the sun.

One concept that can be useful in shifting perception is the idea of "biological" versus "chronological" age. Our chronological age is immutable, but our biological age—how our body functions relative to an average person of our chronological age—can be influenced by lifestyle choices, environment, and yes, attitude.

There's also a community aspect to perception. Cultures that revere the elderly, like some of those in the Blue Zones—areas in the world where people live disproportionately longer—tend to have citizens with more positive attitudes towards aging. Embedding ourselves in communities that value age can bolster our sense of worth and purpose.

Another piece of the puzzle is stress management. Chronic stress can accelerate the aging process at a cellular level, a phenomenon we'll tackle more in-depth later on. Suffice it to say, a mindset that can manage and mitigate stress holds the key to tempering the aging process.

And then there's the role of humor and laughter in perception. Laughing is like an internal workout that reduces stress hormones and increases immune cells. It's quite profound how a hearty laugh can recalibrate our perception of the moment, lifting us out of the trench of age-related worries.

The idea that we can influence our longevity by adjusting our perception of age is empowering. It suggest that there's more room for maneuver than we might've initially thought. It paints a picture of aging not as a downward spiral, but as a spectrum of possibilities.

Maintaining a youthful perception of age can be a self-fulfilling prophecy. When we believe we have the power to influence our health destiny, we're more likely to take the actions necessary to bring that belief to life. As we move through this guide, we'll explore the various facets of aging and longevity. With each new strategy and piece of information, see it as a tool not just for your physical well-being, but for shaping how you perceive and experience age.

Maintaining a Youthful Mindset While the prior sections have adeptly tackled the biological and psychological intricacies of aging, it's pivotal to zero in on the mental frameworks that contribute to a youthful essence. A sprightly mindset isn't just a nice-to-have; it's a cornerstone for those aiming to navigate the labyrinth of longevity with grace and vivacity. The neural pathways in our craniums are malleable, eternally ripe for forging new connections that combat the encroachment of years.

Let's talk about curiosity. Remember when you were a child, and every day brimmed with questions? "Why is the sky blue?" "What makes the grass grow?" Children view the world with wonder because everything is fresh and intriguing. As adults, we sometimes let that curiosity wane, but the truth is, nurturing it keeps our minds engaged and young. So, make it a point to learn something new regularly. It could be as complex as a new language or as simple as a cooking technique. It's less about the what and more about the act of learning itself.

Flexibility in thought is as vital as flexibility in the body. We're talking cognitive suppleness here. A youthful mind adapts, bends, and sometimes even flips perspectives with the ease of a gymnast. Engage in stimulating discussions, entertain contrarian views, and revel in the intellectual jousting that keeps the mind sharp and open.

Positivity could arguably be the elixir of mental youth. It's not about donning rose-colored glasses to view the world but rather choosing to focus on what uplifts rather than what drags down. It's a resilience in the face of setbacks and a capacity to view challenges as opportunities rather than insurmountable barriers. They say laughter is the best medicine, and when it comes to maintaining a youthful spirit, it can be a potent antidote to the wear and tear of time.

Now, let's dip our toes into the fountain of social connectivity. It's no secret that relationships can be complex, but they're also incredibly enriching and play a critical role in keeping your mindset fresh. It's about variety—the young, the old, and everyone in between—connecting across generations and life experiences. Each person you meet can teach you something new, can offer a unique perspective that keeps your mindset from ever growing old.

Then there's the pursuit of passion. Ah, to be zealous about something—anything—is to infuse life with perpetual youthfulness. Passions ignite a fervent energy, a spark that fuels a sense of purpose and excitement. When you invest time in activities that you love, whether they're artistic expressions or sports endeavors, you signal to both body and mind that age is truly just a number.

While discussing passions, one can't omit the importance of goal-setting—a compass that directs your youthful energies towards new horizons. Setting and achieving goals fosters a sense of accomplishment and progress, but don't let these aims stagnate. Regularly revisiting and revising goals keeps them fresh and keeps you motivated and mentally nimble.

But what of resilience? A youthful mindset isn't synonymous with naiveté; it's tempered with the wisdom of experience. Resilience is born from life's trials and tribulations and from understanding that setbacks are not permanent. A resilient mind bounces back, ready to approach life with renewed vigor and a lesson learned.

Playfulness, an often-underestimated mental attribute, deserves a standing ovation. Ever noticed how play is the work of children? Play isn't frivolous; it's a critical exercise in creativity and stress relief. So, integrate play into your daily rituals. A game of charades, an evening of board games, or a playful banter—each are small acts that can inject a dose of youthful joy into your life.

Adventurousness should not be left in the bygones of youth either. The willingness to take risks, to step out of comfort zones, and to explore uncharted territories keeps the thrill of living alive. Be it trying a new restaurant, traveling to an unknown destination, or simply changing your routine—embrace opportunities for adventure to keep your spirit soaring.

Let's not overlook the value of self-reflection. Introspection is a tool for growth—a mirror reflecting back not only the years lived but the depth of those years. Dedicating time for self-reflection encourages self-awareness and personal development. It's about examining life's mosaic and appreciating how each piece, whether bright or somber, contributes to your timeless narrative.

Community involvement also plays a chapter in the book of youthful living. Contributing to the fabric of society can involve mentoring the young, volunteering, or simply engaging in community events. Such engagement not only broadens your social network but also reinforces a sense of purpose and connection, which, in turn, nurtures a youthful outlook.

Mindfulness, though addressed thoroughly in a later chapter, bears mentioning here given its considerable influence on maintaining a youthful disposition. Mindfulness is witnessing the present without judgment—an acceptance that can bring tranquility and a sense of everlasting nowness. It's an appreciation for the moment, which paradoxically, keeps one from becoming mired in the past or fretting over the future.

Finally, in this chorus of youthful strategies, we must touch upon adaptability. It's about evolving with the times, embracing new technologies, and staying relevant. It's recognizing that change is not just inevitable; it's desirable. Adaptability ensures that you are not left behind, but rather marching—or better yet, dancing—along with the forward beat of time.

In closing, crafting a youthful mindset isn't so much about reclaiming what was, but rather about cultivating an attitude that is resilient, adaptive, and vibrant regardless of the chronological tally. It's about engaging with life on all fronts—intellectually, emotionally, and socially to weave a rich, colorful tapestry that celebrates every stage of existence with equal fervor. Remember, the mind is an exquisite garden—tend to it, and it will flourish across all seasons of life.

Chapter 3:
Nutrition for Longevity

As we pivot from the mental landscapes that shape our experience of aging in Chapter 2, the focus now crystalizes on the tangible, on the fuel that propels us through our years—nutrition. Imagine your body as an intricate machine; what we ingest acts as the oil, the nuts and bolts that keep it humming smoothly into the future. The quest for longevity doesn't hinge on some elusive elixir; it's woven into the very fibers of the foods we choose. You're probably aware that a well-balanced diet is key, but let's dig into the nitty-gritty—those select nutrients that have taken a stance against the sands of time, the superhero superfoods that punch well above their weight when it comes to anti-aging. And it's not just about what to eat, but how these fits into broader dietary patterns that cultures around the globe have been whispering about for centuries. We're not talking about trend diets that flare and fade but about sustainable, enjoyable eating habits that could add not just years to your life, but better yet, life to your years. So, let's dive into the core of what can make your diet a bastion of youthfulness, ensuring every bite is a step toward longevity.

Essential Nutrients for Anti-Aging We've discussed the labyrinth of longevity, the mechanics of our biological clock, and the profound effect our mental state has on our aging journey. Let's now shift our focus towards what we can proactively put into our bodies to slow down the hands of time —— the fundamental vitamins, minerals, and nutrients that give us not just life, but a vibrantly aging life. These molecular magicians have the power to nudge our cells away from the brink of senescence and keep our systems humming along smoothly.

Let's first talk vitamins; to age like a fine wine, one cannot ignore the pivotal role of Vitamin D. Aptly nicknamed the 'sunshine vitamin,' this fat-soluble essential helps maintain bone density and immune function, two areas that can be compromised as we age. Spending time outdoors is great but if you can't, consider a supplement, especially in those less sunny months.

Next up, Omega-3 fatty acids, the suave diplomats of the fat world, mediating inflammatory responses and keeping your heart and brain in a state of zen-like calm. Find them in abundance in fatty fish, walnuts, and chia seeds, or if you're not into those, fish oil supplements can be your go-to. They're renowned for their beneficial role in cardiovascular health, rheumatoid arthritis, and even depression, all conditions that tend to become more prevalent as we mark more birthdays.

We can't ignore antioxidants. Imagine them as the body's personal security detail, neutralizing free radicals that can cause oxidative stress, which is akin to biological rusting, speeding up aging. Vitamins C and E are the poster children for antioxidants. Oranges, kiwis, and bell peppers for C; almonds, spinach, and avocados for E, are all excellent reservoirs of youthfulness.

As for minerals, let's chat about calcium. You need strong bones to carry you through the endless dance of life, and calcium is the lead partner. Dairy products are well-known sources, but you've got options in kale, almonds, and fortified plant milks for those seeking plant-based alternatives. Pair your calcium intake with Vitamin D for maximum absorption. Think of it as a pas de deux that keeps osteoporosis at bay.

Zinc should be on your radar too. It's like the unsung hero in the anti-aging tale, supporting immune function and playing a crucial role in wound healing, DNA synthesis, and cell division. A dance with legumes, seeds, and nuts ensures that your body's zinc concerto plays on without missing a beat.

Magnesium might not always be in the limelight, but it's essential for over 300 biochemical reactions in the body, including energy production, which can often wane as we age. Make sure to invite green leafy vegetables, whole grains, and nuts to your daily nutrient feast to keep your energy levels up and running.

Fiber might seem like the boring guest at the nutritional party, but it's one you don't want to miss out on. It keeps your digestive system in tip-top shape, battles cholesterol, and helps regulate blood sugar. Aging might slow some aspects of your physiology, but your gut doesn't have to be one of them. Whole grains, vegetables, and fruits are your go-to fiber friends.

Remember amino acids? They're the building blocks of protein, vital for maintaining muscle mass and strength, which decline as we age, leading to frailty and reduced mobility. Animal products are packed with all the essential amino acids, but for those walking the green path, combining a variety of plant-based proteins can be just as effective.

Lest we forget, hydration. Water might not be a 'nutrient' by classical terms, but it's the medium through which all nutrients travel in our body. Maintaining adequate hydration is tantamount to keeping a well-oiled machine.

Coenzyme Q10 (CoQ10) is another mighty yet underappreciated molecule when talking longevity. It's like your cells' spark plug, critical for energy production. As we age, our bodies produce less CoQ10, which means incorporating foods like organ meats, fatty fish, and whole grains or opting for supplements can give our cell's energy production the jump-start it may need.

Moving on, let's not forget about our friendly bacteria. Probiotics are crucial for a healthy gut microbiome, which in turn is linked to a robust immune system and a decreased risk of chronic diseases. Incorporate fermented foods like yogurt, kefir, and kombucha to support your internal ecosystem.

Selenium is one powerful mineral, a cog in the antioxidant machinery of your body, safeguarding your cells from damage. Found in Brazil nuts, seafood, and grains, introduce this neutralizer to your diet, and it just might provide a protective shield against certain cancers and thyroid disease.

Finally, fluidity in our connective tissues decreases with age, but sulfur-containing nutrients like chondroitin and glucosamine support joint health. These nutrients often come in supplement form and can be the internal lubricant that keeps you moving and grooving.

Ingesting a rainbow of nutrients doesn't guarantee immortality, but it certainly stacks the deck in favor of vibrant health. We've only scratched the surface here, and our adventure in the nutritional landscape continues. From here, we will delve into the nurturing world of superfoods and their anti-aging prowess, but keep this nutrient treasure map close — it's a blueprint to a thriving body and a resilient spirit as the years advance.

Superfoods and Their Anti-Aging Properties As we turn the pages from nutrition fundamentals and sail smoothly into the heart of what fuels our body's resilience against time, let's dive into the world of superfoods. These are not magical substances, but they harness a magnificent tapestry of nutrients that fortify our systems in the silent war against aging.

Superfoods burst with antioxidants, the valiant knights in our battle to keep cellular damage at bay. Picture antioxidants as your body's personal defense force, scavenging harmful free radicals generated by everyday living and environmental stressors, and effectively neutralizing their potential damage.

Take blueberries, for instance. These small but mighty fruits pack a punch of anthocyanins, potent antioxidants which not only give them their vibrant color but also confer benefits such as enhanced brain health and improved memory function. Consistent research suggests that incorporating blueberries into your diet could be a delicious strategy to slow cognitive decline.

Next, there's the omega-3 powerhouse, the wild-caught salmon. Omega-3 fatty acids are not newcomers to the anti-aging scene, revered for their anti-inflammatory properties. But how do they work? They gracefully integrate into your cell membranes, improving cellular health and communication. A well-running cellular network equals a body that ages like fine wine – slowly and splendidly.

Chia seeds make their mark too. These tiny treasures are dense with fiber, protein, omega-3s, and various micronutrients. Their capacity to absorb water and expand can keep you feeling full and curb those cravings that might lead to less beneficial eating habits. After all, maintaining a healthy weight is a crucial act in the saga of aging gracefully.

Then there's the often-hailed kale. This leafy green is swarming with vitamins A, K, C, and numerous minerals. It's not just a trendy salad base; it's a cruciferous crusader in promoting healthy skin and bones and supporting liver function for detoxification processes that our body increasingly craves as we amass more candles on our birthday cakes.

Let's not ignore the sulforaphane-brimming broccoli. Sulforaphane is a compound believed to have potent anti-cancer properties by enhancing detoxification and protecting against oxidative stress. Regularly munching on broccoli might just give your cells that extra armor they need to withstand the test of time.

Almonds shine in the superfood spotlight as well. These nuts are a good source of vitamin E, an antioxidant that's crucial for skin health – acting as a natural sunblock and helping skin retain its natural moisture balance. Here's a little secret: A healthy, radiant skin often reflects the wellness within.

Green tea slides in with catechins, powerful antioxidants that can safeguard your cells from the ruthless invasion of aging. It may be a simple addition to your day, but its effects are far from simplistic. By potentially lowering the risk of heart disease and cancer, this warm, soothing beverage stands tall as a health elixir.

Not to be overshadowed are turmeric's golden hues, the root renowned for its active ingredient, curcumin. Curcumin's anti-inflammatory talents are well-suited to fight chronic inflammation, a sly villain in the aging narrative. It's a spice that not only adds color to your curry but also zest to your years.

Avocados are the creamy gifts from nature that offer monounsaturated fats. These fats are heart-healthy and help maintain the skin's vitality and elasticity. Moreover, substances such as xanthophylls in avocados have been observed to support eye health, serving as a natural defense against age-related macular degeneration.

Then there's the dark chocolate, yes chocolate. When it contains a high cocoa content, it comes loaded with flavanols that may boost brain function, protect your skin against the sun, and keep your heart running smoothly. Indulge sensibly, and chocolate can be your indulgence with a purpose.

The humble garlic, while feared for its social side effects, is truly a giant in the realms of anti-aging. Its active compound, allicin, is a seldom sung hero that can help control blood pressure and work wonders on your immune system, fortifying your disease-fighting potential.

We must not forget about nuts and seeds as a whole. These small but densely nutritious snacks are high in healthy fats and proteins, which are essential for repairing wear and tear throughout the body. They're snacks that keep you young, healthy, and capable of facing the stressors of life head-on.

Finally, the red wine in moderation joins the superfood array with resveratrol, a polyphenol promising to support heart health and potentially mimic some benefits of calorie restriction – one of the few strategies scientifically shown to extend life span. Enjoy your glass judiciously, and it's not just the present moment that cheers; your future self may too.

As these superfoods take the stage, it's essential to recognize that they're most potent when part of a balanced and diverse diet. Their anti-aging properties don't arise from solitary consumption but from a symphony played in harmony with other nutrients and lifestyle factors. They're not a panacea, but they're powerful allies on your journey to a life well-lived and well-extended.

So next time you find yourself navigating your kitchen or pacing the aisles of your local grocery store, ponder the potency of these superfoods in your anti-aging arsenal. It's about making smart, flavorful choices that not only tickle your palate but also nurture your body's resilience against the ticking clock. Take charge of your health, one supercharged bite at a time.

Dietary Patterns for a Longer Life In our pursuit of a timeline dotted with an abundance of candles, let's talk about the fuel we're putting in our tanks. There's an old saying that you can't outrun a bad diet, and when it comes to longevity, tacking on those extra years isn't just about moving more—it's equally, if not more, about what's on your plate. We've delved into superfoods and nutrients in previous chapters, but now it's time to weave those threads into a tapestry of dietary patterns that claim a stake in the land of longevity.

Imagine walking through a market where baskets overflow with deep-colored berries, nuts that seem to whisper tales of ancient trees, and greens so vibrant they almost hum with life. These aren't mere ingredients; they're cornerstones of a life-extending feast. But, let's pivot from the poetic and get down to the brass tacks—what exactly are the dietary patterns that those revered for their longer lives follow?

The Mediterranean diet gets plenty of applause, and it's not without merit. Picture this: a dietary symphony starring fruits, vegetables, whole grains, lean proteins, and a love affair with olive oil. It's a diet that sings to the rhythm of heart health and waltzes with the promise of longevity. Numerous studies vouch for its effectiveness in keeping chronic diseases at bay, and lest we forget, it also plays a cameo in the longevity Hotspots—areas known as Blue Zones.

Blue Zones: ever heard of them? These are pockets around the world where people live alarmingly longer than average. And when we peek into their kitchens, we notice a pattern akin to the Mediterranean diet, but with local twists. For instance, Okinawans from Japan cherish their sweet potatoes, Sardinians have a penchant for sourdough bread, and Ikarians thrive on a splash of red wine. It's not about copying and pasting a diet; it's about adapting the essence, the ethos of eating for a long, fulfilling life.

Take plant-based diets—they're gaining attention faster than a new celebrity diet, but with much sturdier legs to stand on. Broccoli and its leafy companions are more than sides; they're headliners in a diet that starves inflammations and malignancies while feeding cellular renewal.

Let's not pretend it's an easy switch if you're accustomed to a different eating script, but the teeming evidence in favor of plants is compelling enough to consider a scene change.

Now, before meat lovers feel cornered, it's not about banishing animal protein to the pages of history. It's about portion sizes and frequencies, about embracing meats as a part of the meal, not the meal itself. Lean cuts, fish rich in omega-3's, and poultry without the skin strutting in moderation—that's the balancing act seen in longevity-heralding diets.

Intermittent fasting has its chapter too. Like a plot twist in a good novel, the idea of skipping meals, albeit strategically, may add years to your life. By periodically pushing the pause button on eating, we're tossing our bodies a challenge, and it's a challenge that might just rev up those living engines to ward off age-related decline.

We'd be remiss not to mention the nuts and bolts—literally, nuts are powerhouse snacks. They're like nature's own vitamin pills but with better packaging. Walnuts, almonds, pistachios—they're not just for holiday platters; they're for everyday longevity. And the bolts? Those are your seeds: flax, chia, and hemp sprinkled over meals for a fibrous, Omega-rich crunch.

The tapestry of a longevity diet is also woven with the threads of hydration. While not a "food" per se, water is the fluid foundation of life, playing a role in nearly every bodily function. And teas, especially green tea, steeped in antioxidants, are like an internal spa for your cells.

So, what's the lowdown on the sweets and treats? Dark chocolate sneaks under the tapestry as a darling of indulgence that can still play nice with longevity, thanks to its flavonoids. The lesson? A little bit of what you fancy does you good, as long as it's just a bit.

Convenience food—the nemesis to our longevity saga. Store-bought meals and fast-food joints might be easy on time, but they're harsh on our life's timeline. They're usually rife with the sort of fats our bodies could do without, loaded with salt and conversing with calories that bring little to the table, nutrition-wise.

This brings us to diversity, not just in life experiences, but on your plate. A colorful platter means a wider array of nutrients, each with its role to play in maintaining your body's vitality. Don't get stuck in a dietary monochrome; embrace the rainbow of fruits and vegetables, and revel in the different strokes of dietary colors.

Lastly, the pacing of your meals also co-authors the story of your longevity. Eating mindfully, savoring each bite, not just for the flavor but for the life it's fueling, can recalibrate the way your body processes food. Slowing down at the dining table isn't just a social affair; it's a personal investment in your longevity account.

Armed with these patterns and considering the uniqueness of your own life's script, personalization is key. What works for one may not work for another, but the blueprint of a longevity diet is clear—it's rich in plants, friendly to the heart, and it veers away from the processed path.

In wrapping this up, let's remind ourselves that the pursuit of a longer life isn't merely about adding years to the timeline. It's about enriching those years with quality, vitality, and zest. It's not just about living longer; it's about thriving every step of the way. As we knit the next chapters, keep these dietary patterns in your culinary script—they're the secret to not just a longer life, but a splendid journey toward it.

Chapter 4:
The Hydration Factor

As we pivot from the complex tapestry of nutritional essentials that form our dietary defense against the tick-tock of time, let's dive into the tides of the Hydration Factor. Water, you see, isn't just the essence of wetness—it's the essence of youth. Think of a plant, deprived of moisture, wilting away. Not a bad metaphor for what happens to our cells without proper hydration, which plays a starring role in maintaining cellular integrity and facilitating countless physiological processes. But hydration is no simple matter of eight glasses a day. It's about timing, purity, and the interplay with other nutrients that multiply its youth-preserving powers. The elixir of life is right at your fingertips, yet so often overlooked in its simplicity and readily available abundance. A sip here, a glass there, and we sustain the vitality of every cell, buoy the skin's suppleness, and keep the systems that cleanse and energize us whirring. Thirst isn't just a signal, it's a harbinger—a nudge from within gently reminding us that to sustain the zest and vivacity, one must never overlook the humble majesty of a hydrating quaff.

Water and Aging: The Undeniable Connection As we delve into the critical role of hydration, we're treading on the shores of a profound truth that echoes through our biology. Our bodies are vast oceans wrapped in skin, ever so dependent on the nurturing ebb and flow of water.

Since the dawn of time, water has been a symbol of life – and rightly so. Within the intricate workings of our bodies, water is the silent orchestrator of countless biochemical symphonies. It's not just about quenching thirst or taking the edge off a dry mouth; water is pivotal for maintaining our physiological processes in a state of harmony.

Imagine your cells as bustling cities, with water as the primary mode of transport in and out of them. It carries in nutrients and shuttles out waste, a relentless cycle that keeps our cells functioning at their peak. The simple act of drinking water is akin to maintaining the roads and canals within these cities – neglect leads to congestion and breakdown, which over time can take a toll on the entire organism.

Metabolism, often talked about in the context of weight management, hinges heavily on our hydration status. Water acts as the medium for metabolic reactions, aiding in the conversion of food into energy. It's a bit like the oil that keeps an engine running smoothly. Without sufficient water, our metabolism can stutter and stall, a deficit that may not only affect our waistlines but also our energy levels and overall vitality.

As we age, our body's water content naturally diminishes. This decline in cellular hydration can lead to a myriad of issues; from reduced elasticity in the skin, signaling the outward signs of aging, to more profound internal effects such as decreased kidney function and cognitive decline.

Joint health, too, is at the mercy of our hydration habits. Those creaks and groans that become more pronounced with age are partly due to the drying out of our synovial fluid – the lubricant that allows our joints to move smoothly. Regular hydration keeps this fluid at its optimal viscosity, ensuring that our movements remain as fluid as they were in younger years.

Speaking of cognition, let's not overlook the brain's affair with hydration. A dehydrated mind is akin to a riverbed cracked and parched under a scorching sun – its thought streams become sluggish and its cognitive functions, less sharp. Mental clarity and concentration can decline with dehydration, and over time, staying well-hydrated can act as a buffer against the cognitive erosion that comes with aging.

But it's not just about keeping enough water flowing through our bodies; quality matters too. The drinking water that fills our glasses should be clean and rich in minerals, offering us the building blocks for maintaining a robust physique as the years tick by.

One could wonder, how much water is enough to stave off the creeping dryness of age? While the "eight glasses a day" adage is a familiar refrain, the truth is more nuanced. Our water needs are as individual as our fingerprints, fluctuating with our lifestyle, the climate we live in, and our dietary choices.

It might seem a daunting task to keep track of something as ubiquitous as water consumption, but herein lies a potent strategy in the art of aging gracefully. Monitoring one's water intake and responding to the body's cues for hydration is as much a pillar of longevity as any sophisticated diet or rigorous exercise regimen.

Also, let's not forget that water isn't just in our cups and bottles. It's present in abundant amounts in fruits and vegetables, a natural reservoir of hydration and nutrients. These foods offer a two-fold benefit for aging gracefully: they are sources of essential vitamins and antioxidants, while their high water content contributes significantly to our daily water intake.

The effects of dehydration can often masquerade as other ailments, like hunger or fatigue. The solution can be as simple as a glass of water, yet so often, it's overlooked. As we venture into our golden years, the regular act of hydrating can pull back the curtain on these masqueraders, revealing a more vibrant, energetic self.

This connection between water and aging is as clear as a pristine spring. Our bodies may carry the wisdom of years, but our cells still clamor for the life-giving essence of water. It's a basic need that becomes ever more critical as we navigate the tides of time.

To harness the full potential of water in the context of aging, it's not about overhauling one's entire lifestyle overnight. It's about making small, sustainable shifts – choosing water over a soda, enjoying a juicy piece of fruit, or starting the morning with a tall glass of water to awaken the senses and hydrate the body from its overnight rest.

As we continue this discourse, we must remember that water is not a panacea. It is, however, a fundamental strand in the tapestry of aging well. Keeping our internal seas replenished is a simple yet forceful affirmation of life, a daily act of self-care that reverberates through the years, helping us to maintain resilience, vitality, and grace as the chapters of our life unfold.

Optimal Hydration Strategies As we've explored the integral role water plays in aging, let's now turn to the art of hydration – a dance between not just drinking water, but doing so effectively. Consider it a strategic move within the grand game of promoting longevity. So, what does optimal hydration look like as we age? Let's dive into the quenching details.

In the primordial quest for the elixir of life, one might be surprised to find that water holds the closest resemblance. Proper hydration facilitates countless bodily functions – from cellular renewal to toxin elimination. Recall those mornings when you've woken up feeling less than refreshed; often, a glass of water can do more than just wet your whistle – it can energetically kick-start your day.

The reality is that our sensation of thirst becomes less acute as we age. Thus, the strategy shifts from merely responding to our bodies' pleas for hydration to preventing dehydration proactively. Start by setting consistent reminders to drink water throughout the day. Smartphones or even a simple kitchen timer can serve as an ally in this mission.

Customizing your intake is crucial, too. Contrary to popular belief, that age-old advice of eight glasses a day isn't a one-size-fits-all solution. Factors like weight, climate, and activity levels dictate our unique hydration needs. Preemptively adjusting your water intake to accommodate exercise sessions or hot weather becomes a winning tactic in maintaining homeostasis.

Fine-tuning further, integrating food with high water content into meals can be a secret weapon. Think cucumbers, bell peppers, and tomatoes, or fruits like watermelon and strawberries. These hydrating foods provide a dual benefit – a marriage of nourishment and water that is especially beneficial for those who find chugging water throughout the day monotonous.

Sometimes, the obstacles in our path to optimal hydration masquerade as the drinks we love. Caffeine and alcohol act as diuretics, often leading us to lose more fluids than we take in. Moderation is the key, and for every cup of coffee or glass of wine, consider following it with an equal amount of water.

When it comes to water quality, don't be deceived by the myth that only bottled water is good for you. Many tap waters are fortified with fluoride and lack the microplastics found in bottled water. However, factors like location and water source can affect purity, so it may be worth investing in a home filtration system to ensure every glass is as beneficial as possible.

The nutritional world often touts the benefits of electrolytes, and rightfully so, as they're vital for hydration. With every sweat session, we strip our bodies of these essential minerals. Replenishing with a balanced electrolyte drink post-workout assists in hydration and helps prevent muscle cramps and fatigue.

But be wary of commercial sports drinks, as they can be teeming with sugars and artificial additives. Instead, look for natural electrolyte sources or consider making your own replenishing beverage with just water, a pinch of salt, and a squeeze of lemon or lime for a refreshing twist that aids in hydration without unnecessary extras.

The temperature of your water also plays a subtle but significant role. While ice-cold water can be invigorating on a warm day, room temperature water is often better absorbed by the body. Warmth encourages vasodilation – an expanding of our vessels – allowing the H_2O to reach its destination more efficiently.

Continuous hydration isn't just a daytime endeavor; it extends into the night. However, balance is important to avoid disrupting sleep with nocturnal trips to the restroom. Aim for a modest intake in the evening and establish a cut-off point a few hours before bedtime to minimize interruption.

For those with a competitive streak, turning hydration into a challenge adds an element of fun. Join forces with friends or family in tracking daily water intake. Not only does it create accountability, but it also fosters a spirit of camaraderie in pursuit of a common goal – staying healthfully hydrated.

Don't forget the power of visual cues. Out of sight can mean out of mind, so keeping a water bottle at your desk, in your car, or in your bag provides a constant physical reminder to take a sip. Investing in a bottle that you find aesthetically pleasing and functional increases the likelihood of it becoming a staple in your daily routine.

Ancillary techniques, such as using apps to log water intake or setting daily goals, can harness the power of technology to keep hydration top of mind. With so many resources at our fingertips, there's no excuse not to keep tabs on our water consumption.

Lastly, listen to your body. Despite decreasing thirst sensitivity with age, other signals can alert us to dehydration. Dry lips, headaches, or fatigue often serve as early warning flags. Staying attuned to these signs can guide your hydration practices to be responsive as well as proactive.

Ultimately, water is our lifeblood, especially as we traverse the age spectrum. Adopting these optimal hydration strategies is less about following strict rules and more about creating a lifestyle that acknowledges the fluidity (pun intended) of our hydration needs over time. Implementing these methods sets a foundation for a more vibrant, youthful existence where every cell in our body can thrive in the symphony of sustained wellness. Drink up – your future self will thank you.

Chapter 5:
Physical Activity and Aging

We've just quenched our thirst with the hydration wisdom of Chapter 4, and now it's time to energize that well-hydrated body with the power of movement. Embracing physical activity as we age isn't just about warding off the rust that time seems intent on applying; it's about rediscovering the vitality that courses through us, no matter the numbers on our birthday cake. This chapter is your gym buddy, encouraging you to harness the magic of endorphins and build strength, flexibility, and balance that defy the years. We're not talking about Herculean feats—just the joys of motion that help keep our cells dancing, our hearts serenading, and our joints celebrating. By integrating tailored exercises with the know-how of your body's rhythms and needs as it matures, you can craft an anti-aging workout plan that feels less like a routine and more like a personal revolution. So let's tie those shoelaces and set the stage for a life where every step, swim, and stretch is a toast to enduring youthfulness.

The Best Exercises for Age-Defying Fitness As we've journeyed through the intricacies of aging, from the biological underpinnings to the nourishment of our cells, let's shift our focus to the linchpin of age-defying vitality: physical activity. Acknowledge this - the fountain of youth isn't a mythical spring; it courses through the very act of movement. So, let's delve into a regimen of the best exercises that promise to keep the years gracefully at bay.

Firstly, cardiovascular exercise is paramount. Engaging in activities like brisk walking, cycling, swimming, or jogging pumps the heart, improves circulation, and can stave off conditions such as heart disease, stroke, and diabetes. But here's the kicker – these aren't merely workouts; they are the rituals that recharge our biological battery. Aim for at least 150 minutes of moderate aerobic activity or 75 minutes of vigorous activity each week to court these benefits.

Now, couple that cardio with strength training. The loss of muscle mass, or sarcopenia, is synonymous with aging. However, lifting weights or using resistance bands reverses this narrative. Not only does it bolster muscle and bone strength, but it's also a crusader against osteoporosis and frailty. A consistent routine, targeting all major muscle groups at least twice a week, can elevate your metabolic rate and turn your body into an efficient energy-burning engine.

Yoga and Pilates emerge as the sculptors of flexibility and balance - qualities that diminish with time but can be marvelously reclaimed. These disciplines enhance core strength, posture, and mental focus. By integrating them into your weekly routine, perhaps through a class or at-home practice, you can foster agility that defies the decades.

Don't underestimate the power of balance exercises, either. Activities such as tai chi, or even simple exercises like standing on one leg, fortify the stabilizing muscles and help prevent falls, a common cause of injury among older adults. The grace of balance is subtle, but it reinforces the very freedom that mobility affords.

Then there's the less celebrated, but no less crucial, practice of stretching. Maintaining range of motion through regular stretching sessions is a lifeline to muscles and joints. It's the difference between moving with ease or stiffness as years march on. Carve out time after workouts or during a calming evening routine to gently extend muscles and embrace the fluidity of movement.

High-Intensity Interval Training (HIIT) might sound daunting, but it's a boon for metabolism and reversing age-related decline in muscle health. This type of training alternates short bursts of intense activity with periods of rest or lower-intensity exercise. With HIIT, you see benefits in a fraction of the time compared to traditional workouts. For the seasoned exerciser, it can catalyze a vibrant aging process.

And let's not overlook functional fitness – exercises that train your muscles to work together, preparing them for daily tasks by simulating common movements. Think squats, lunges, and rotations; movements that mimic reaching, lifting, and bending. These maintain the independence that is so cherished as we age.

Aquatic exercises deserve a special mention. The buoyancy of water supports the body, reducing the strain on joints, making it an ideal medium for age-defying workouts. Swimming, water aerobics, or just walking in water can deliver a full-body workout without wear and tear.

Dance, too, is an underrated gem. It's not just an expression of art; it's a comprehensive exercise that melds aerobic, strength, and flexibility training with balance and coordination. Plus, it's a jubilant way to connect with others, weaving social threads into the fabric of fitness.

Walking is perhaps the most accessible exercise of all and it's loaded with perks. It improves cardiovascular endurance, bolsters bone health, and elevates mood. A brisk daily walk can be the touchstone of a health-centric lifestyle, offering a moment for reflection or companionship.

As you approach your regime, heed this adage: consistency trumps intensity. A moderate, steady approach to fitness, aligned with your body's signals, is more sustainable and rewarding in the long-term than intermittent bouts of extreme exercise.

Moreover, always consult with healthcare professionals before initiating a fitness program, especially if you have pre-existing health conditions. They can guide you towards exercise that complements your unique physiological blueprint.

What's profound about exercise is its ripple effect. Beyond the evident benefits, such as improved endurance and muscle tone, it enhances sleep quality, sharpens cognitive function, and mitigates stress. It's the cornerstone of a vigorous and resilient life, no matter the number of candles on your birthday cake.

Last but not least, track your progress and celebrate your triumphs, no matter how small. Whether it's increased stamina, a new level of flexibility, or simply the feel-good endorphins post-workout - these milestones are your personal accolades in the quest for age-defying fitness.

In closing, remember – while we cannot outpace time, we can certainly jog alongside it with poise. Craft a routine from these varied exercises, and you'll not just add years to your life; you'll infuse life into your years.

Designing Your Personal Anti-Aging Workout Plan can seem like threading a needle in a field of haystacks—rewards are abundant but only when the method clicks perfect with your lifestyle. The aim here isn't to chase an unattainable fountain of youth but to craft a regime that is sustainable, enjoyable, and deeply rejuvenating for your body's unique needs.

Start with pondering what physical activities you naturally enjoy. Is it a solitary, reflective jog in the cool morning air? A fiery Zumba class that leaves a smile plastered to your face? Your workout plan isn't just about longevity; it's about weaving the fabric of joy into your day-to-day life. Moving your body shouldn't be a chore, but a celebration of what it can still accomplish.

Next, balance is the crux. A comprehensive workout plan nudges you out of your comfort zone, but is never punitive. There's merit to mixing strength training with flexibility drills, aerobic exercises with balance-focused routines. Remember, the sinewy might of muscle and the yielding grace of stretched tendons contribute equally to your body's anti-aging symphony.

Progression can't be underscored enough. Start with exercises that pose a fair challenge and gradually augment the difficulty. The philosophy here is to let the body adapt, evolve, and never plateau. It's not chasing after personal records each day but rather, it's about upping the ante just enough to kindle growth.

Consistency weaves the pattern. Random fits and bursts of activity, albeit intense, can't form the cornerstone of a truly age-defying routine. Lock in a time of day, figure out frequency, and then, rain or shine, stick with it. Your body's internal clock will thank you for the regularity.

And while we're on the subject of time, don't let duration intimidate you. Effective workouts don't necessarily demand hours. Science nods at the efficacy of short, intense workouts. The idea is to maintain a vibrant metabolic dance and not wear yourself down to a fatigued, counterproductive stump.

Periodic reassessment is as crucial as the workout itself. It's about tapping into how your body feels in response to your workouts. Does it feel challenged? Energized? If your regimen feels akin to running into a brick wall repeatedly, it's time to reassess. Constantly evolve your fitness plan to match your body's ever-changing capabilities and limitations.

List listening should be your mantra, as in listening to your body. Be attentive to its whispers and don't wait for the screams. A mild discomfort might simply require slight modification, whereas playing through pain can spell a lengthy, unwanted hiatus down the line.

For the older battalion, resistance training deserves a special mention. As bones look towards retreating, weight-bearing exercises remind them there's a battle to be fought. Resistance training, even with light weights, boosts bone density and staves off the brittle whispers of osteoporosis.

Don't underestimate the power of the great outdoors. Sunlight bestows Vitamin D, fresh air dusts off cobwebs in the mind, and the changing scenery keeps monotony at bay. Whenever viable, take your workout outside; let nature's elements play the role of a silent coach.

As you chart your course, remember, your journey is uniquely yours. The internet may parade countless 'cutting-edge' workout formulas, but unless they resonate with you at a core level, they're just abstract blueprints. Pick what fits into your life's puzzle; often, personal intuition trumps conventional wisdom.

Rest should be inked into your plan with the same priority as the workouts. It's during rest that muscles are forged and the body fortifies itself. Skimping on recovery can pull the reins on an otherwise galloping anti-aging steed.

Integration, not isolation, should be the overall approach. Your workout plan can't be walled off from the rest of your life. It should mesh seamlessly with your nutritional choices, sleep patterns, stress levels, and social interactions. It's this integrative approach that reaps the most bountiful harvest when it comes to anti-aging.

Edging towards the endgame, it's not just about penciling workouts into your calendar but also engraining them into your identity. The resolve to remain active and embrace exercise as a daily staple is what eventually separates fleeting fads from enduring triumphs in the anti-aging wars.

As you forge your personal workout plan, imbue it with flexibility. Life will invariably throw curveballs, and your workout plan must have the elasticity to adapt. A rigid regimen is bound to crack, but one that's pliable will sway, survive, and thrive, much like the well-tempered spirit of youth.

And finally, reward yourself for milestones achieved. Celebrating progress, no matter how slight, reinforces the positive loop between mind and muscle. Whether it's a new workout gear or a day of complete rest, these rewards are physical tokens of your commitment to aging not just gracefully but vigorously, actively steering your life towards wellness and longevity.

Chapter 6:
The Importance of Sleep

Just as the right nutrition fuels your days, think of sleep as the essential charge for your body's batteries, without which everything starts to lose its spark. We often wear our 'I'll sleep when I'm dead' badge with a misplaced sense of pride, not understanding that skimping on sleep can make us feel, well, less alive. Dive into the world of slumber, and you'll uncover that sleep isn't just a timeout from our busy lives; it's an active state where restoration and rejuvenation occur, processes especially critical as we age. Sure, your skin might crave that nightly eight-hour treatment, but it's your mind and every cell in your body that reap the anti-aging rewards. Deeper sleep stages untangle the day's mental knots, boost memory consolidation, and repair tissues, setting you up for a brighter morning and a healthier tomorrow, not to mention the impact on metabolic health, hormonal balance, and immune function. If vitality and longevity are what you're after, ignoring sleep is like trying to climb a mountain with no base camp - you simply won't get far. The following pages don't just sing lullabies; they're packed with actionable insights to help you harness the transformative power of sleep, enhancing every facet of your being and gracefully guiding you through your anti-aging journey.

Sleep Patterns and Their Effect on Aging Transitioning smoothly from considering exercises to defy aging in the previous chapter, we now turn our focus to an equally important but often undervalued pillar of longevity: sleep. It's a ubiquitous part of our daily lives, yet the complex relationship between sleep patterns and aging remains a subject ripe for discussion. How we slumber through the night can be as critical to our health as our diet and exercise routines—if not more so.

Sleep is not simply a passive state of rest but a dynamic process that affects our bodies and minds in profound ways. Over the years, research has consistently shown that sleep plays a critical role in restoring and rejuvenating our bodies. It's during these quiet hours that our body repairs damaged cells, consolidates memories, and balances hormones—processes that are integral to aging gracefully.

A lack of quality sleep, on the other hand, can leave us feeling drained and foggy. It can disrupt metabolic processes, imparting an adverse effect on weight management, insulin sensitivity, and cardiovascular health. In the puzzle of aging, fragmented sleep patterns can be like a piece that doesn't quite fit, throwing off the entire picture of health we strive to maintain.

As we age, our sleep architecture—referring to the structure and pattern of our sleep cycles—naturally shifts. You might recall times when staying up late posed no challenge, or when 'sleeping in' was a weekend staple. However, for many, those days recede with time, leaving in their place a tendency for earlier bedtimes and, frustratingly, earlier wake times.

It's not just the hours that change; the quality of sleep undergoes transformation as well. Older adults often experience a decrease in deep, restorative sleep and an increase in nighttime awakenings—disruptions that can impair the body's ability to repair itself. This change in sleep pattern can have a cascade of effects on physical health, from exacerbated chronic conditions to a weakened immune system.

The sleeper's brain isn't just a passive beneficiary of a good night's rest either. During sleep, particularly during rapid eye movement (REM) stages, our brains are hard at work. This is when the brain's custodial services kick into high gear, clearing out toxins including beta-amyloid, a protein associated with the development of Alzheimer's disease. Consistent, high-quality sleep may thus serve as a form of nightly detoxification, critical for maintaining cognitive health as we age.

Is there an optimal amount of sleep for anti-aging? Studies are hinting at a "sweet spot" not too different from the oft-touted seven to eight hours per night. Skimping on sleep consistently can push our bodies into a state of stress, invoking inflammatory responses and oxidative damage—both players in the aging process. Too much sleep isn't ideal either, potentially signaling underlying health issues or contributing to a sedentary lifestyle, which comes with its own aging accelerants.

Then there's the issue of chronotypes, the natural inclination for some of us to be morning larks or night owls. Respecting our individual chronotype can be instrumental in achieving high-quality sleep. Your genes play a role in your natural sleep-wake cycle, and fighting against it may cause hormonal imbalances and circadian rhythm disruptions that crack the spine of your wellbeing.

The cultural phenomenon of "burning the midnight oil" risks not just immediate tiredness but also long-term health concerns. Artificial light, especially the blue light emanating from screens, can throw off our circadian rhythms, tricking our brains into thinking it's still daylight long after the sun has set. This confusion can delay the production of melatonin, the sleep hormone, reducing sleep quality and potentially accelerating aging.

Dietary choices also weave their way into our nocturnal tapestry. Caffeine, alcohol, and heavy meals close to bedtime can all interrupt the quality of sleep. Moreover, the interplay between diet, sleep, and aging is complex and bidirectional—poor sleep can spark cravings for less-than-healthy foods, which can then snowball into more sleep issues. Establishing better sleep hygiene can thus go hand-in-hand with a healthier diet.

What about naps, those short bursts of sleep that can either refresh or disrupt? While napping can be beneficial, especially as we get older, timing their length and frequency is key. Long or irregular napping can interfere with nighttime sleep patterns and may not offer the restorative benefits of a full night's sleep, thereby potentially impacting the aging process.

And it's not just nighttime when sleep holds sway over our aging; it's during the day too. Regular physical activity can promote better sleep quality, creating a virtuous cycle that enhances overall health and longevity. Conversely, a sedentary lifestyle can have a detrimental impact on sleep quality and duration, thereby influencing the aging process adversely.

In the upcoming section, we delve deeper into strategies to improve sleep quality. But for now, let's sit with the recognition that understanding and optimizing our sleep patterns is an indispensable strategy in our anti-aging toolkit.

It's clear then, the contours of our sleep are etched deeply into the fabric of how we age. From the timing to the amount, the quality to the consistency, every aspect of our slumber is intertwined with the vitality of our twilight years. As we forge onward in our journey of aging with intention and grace, let us not forget the silent, yet powerful ally that is a good night's rest.

Strategies for Improved Sleep Quality Leaping from understanding the impact of sleep on aging, it's time to arm you with strategies to enhance those precious hours of slumber. As we venture into the twilight of our years, our sleep patterns take a hit, becoming more fragmented and less deep. Yet, consistent, restorative sleep is a pillar of longevity, and mastering it can have you greeting each morning with vigor.

The sanctity of the sleep environment is paramount. Your bedroom should be a temple dedicated to rest. Keep it cool, dark, and quiet. Blackout curtains can ward off intrusive light, and the right temperature, slightly on the cooler side, beckons your body to sleep. If silence isn't golden due to urban clamor or a partner's snoring symphony, consider a white noise machine to mask the cacophony.

Regularizing your sleep schedule sets your internal clock to predictability. Strive to wake up and go to bed at the same times daily, yes, even on weekends. Your body's circadian rhythms align, bolstering sleep quality and continuity. This consistency can be the stabilizing force your sleep craves as you age.

Nutritional harmony plays a lilting tune in this sleep symphony. Avoid heavy meals and alcohol close to bedtime; they're marauders of rest, disrupting the architecture of your sleep. Meanwhile, caffeine is a formidable foe to slumber, and its effects can linger. Steering clear of it post-afternoon helps secure uninterrupted sleep.

Daylight is a conductor of your biological rhythms. Exposure to natural light, especially in the morning, reinforces your body's daytime wakefulness, priming you for better sleep at night. It's the natural world's way of setting your internal rhythms in sync with the environment.

Physical activity is a timeless ally; weaving exercise into your day can consolidate nighttime sleep. However, timing is crucial. Too close to bedtime, and the resultant endorphin release can keep you counting sheep far longer than you'd like. Aim for at least a few hours' buffer before bed to allow your body to unwind and relax.

A pre-slumber ritual is like a familiar lullaby. It might involve dimming lights, sipping chamomile tea, or reading a book. This transition period signals to your body that it's time to wind down, easing the transition from wakefulness to sleep.

Let's not forget the physical mattress and pillows you entrust with your nocturnal repose. Invest in their quality. A supportive mattress and pillows catering to your preferred sleeping position can banish aches and enhance the depth of your sleep.

Monitor your liquid intake as evening falls; too much fluid can lead to nocturnal interruptions. Staying hydrated is important, but balance is key. Aim to front-load your fluid intake earlier in the day and taper as bedtime approaches.

Despite our best efforts, stress snakes into our lives, and it's a notorious thief of sleep. Developing stress-management techniques can help. From deep-breathing exercises to progressive muscle relaxation or mindfulness, these practices can ease the mind and reduce the time it takes to fall asleep.

If you're grappling with persistent sleep trouble, perhaps it's time for a sleep diary. Tracking your sleep patterns and habits can uncover hidden disruptors. Share this diary with a healthcare professional for personalized insights and solutions.

Technology's blue light is an insidious sleep saboteur. It mimics daylight, tricking your brain into daylight mode. Power down those screens ideally two hours before bed, allowing your melatonin to crest naturally, cueing your body for sleep.

Sometimes, ambiance is everything. Enfold your senses in calming scents, such as lavender, to usher in tranquility. While the evidence on their effectiveness varies, many swear by aromatherapy's power to relax the mind and soul, preparing both for restful sleep.

Lastly, if worries and to-dos are carouseling in your head, scribe them. Penning your thoughts can offload them from your mind, making space for serenity and, ultimately, sleep.

Consider these strategies as individual threads in a tapestry. Not every thread will resonate with every soul, but woven together with care, they can form your bespoke blanket of better sleep. The goal is to tailor these tactics to your life rhythm, aligning them in harmony with your unique sleep needs.

As daylight dims and stars emerge, you can now approach bedtime with confidence, armed with strategies to foster deep, restorative slumber. Embrace them as not just tools for longevity but as nightly companions on your journey to a vibrant and youthful tomorrow.

Chapter 7:
Stress Management Techniques

As we pivot from the revitalizing power of sleep discussed in the previous chapter, let's dive into the invigorating world of stress management. It's no secret that stress is a stealthy ager, stealthily sneaking up and leaving its mark on our well-being, but here's the good news: we can take the reins back. Consider this a toolkit, chock-full of stress-busting techniques to not just handle life's pressures but to thrive in spite of them. You'll learn how to recognize the sneaky symptoms of stress that often go unnoticed until they manifest in more significant health issues. Think of these strategies as your personal stress-deflecting armor—effective practices that can be seamlessly woven into your daily routine, fortifying your resilience against the potentially aging effects of stress. It's about transforming your response to life's inevitable challenges, using techniques grounded in science, yet simple enough to integrate into your bustling life. With the right approach, managing stress becomes less about avoidance and more about robust engagement, fostering a life replete with vitality, and leading you ever closer to that enviable fountain of youth.

Understanding the Impact of Stress on Aging You've marveled at the science of aging, grappled with the complexities of sleep, and fine-tuned your diet for longevity. But there's a silent infiltrator that could be aging you faster than you think: stress. The chameleon of the modern age, stress is often masked behind busy schedules and high-pressure lifestyles. Yet, its effects are far from invisible especially when it comes to how you age.

Imagine stress as an incessant drip on the metal of your resilience—over time, it can corrode even the strongest of defenses. This isn't poetic scaremongering; there's strong scientific evidence to show that chronic stress can promote biological aging, nudging your cells to age prematurely. It's as though stress has its fingers on the fast-forward button of life's remote control.

To grasp how stress is capable of such shenanigans, let's talk telomeres, those nifty little caps at the ends of chromosomes that protect our genetic material. Think of them as the plastic tips on shoelaces, keeping the lace intact. Every time a cell divides, telomeres shorten slightly until—after many divisions—they're too short to protect the chromosomes, and the cell can no longer regenerate. It's a natural part of aging; but here's the rub: stress can accelerate telomere shortening.

Why does this matter? Telomeres might just be microscopic, but their length is linked to an array of age-related diseases. Shorter telomeres have been associated with cardiovascular disease, type 2 diabetes, and osteoporosis, among other health issues. So stress, by speeding up the deterioration of these little guardians, could be paving a shortcut to these conditions.

Cortisol, known as the 'stress hormone,' goes up when we're in 'fight or flight' mode. Handy for running away from tigers, not so handy for our health when the level persists long after the perceived threat has gone. Prolonged high cortisol levels wreak havoc on our bodies, suppressing the immune system, increasing blood pressure, and contributing to the buildup of abdominal fat—a marker associated with increased risk of heart disease and insulin resistance.

Furthermore, stress isn't just about molecules and hormones—it has tangible effects on your daily behavior. It can disrupt your sleep, lead to poor eating habits, reduce your motivation to exercise, and even cause you to age in appearance faster than you'd expect. The stereotypes of gray hair from worry or stress lines etching in aren't completely unfounded.

Now, let's connect the dots between psychological stress and longevity. Emotions like anxiety and depression can dampen your will to maintain those healthful habits crucial for a long life. An overwhelmed mind is less likely to choose a nutritious salad over comfort food, or lace up for a refreshing run over collapsing on the couch. Over time, these choices accumulate, like plaque on the arteries of our well-being.

But there's good news buried amid the gloom. Stress, despite its pervasive nature, isn't a life sentence of accelerated decline. The brain is remarkable, showing an enviable plasticity and in those twists and turns of neurons and synapses, there lie strategies waiting to be tapped for managing stress.

The first step is acknowledging stress. You can't manage what you don't measure or accept. This acknowledgment isn't about assigning blame; it's about empowering you to take back control. From laid-back attitudes to mindful practices, employing a variety of strategies can blunt the cutting edge of stress, buffering your body from its aging effects.

Destressing techniques range from the traditional, like meditation and yoga, to the contemporary, like 'digital detoxes' and pet therapy. By integrating such practices into your daily routine, you can mitigate the damaging effects stress has on your body and, by extension, your aging process.

Remember, it's not about purging stress entirely—some stress is helpful. It keeps us sharp, motivated, and even healthy in the right amounts. It's the chronic, unyielding stress that's detrimental. The aim then is to navigate a path through life that moderates stress to a constructive level rather than letting it become destructive.

By understanding the mechanisms behind the impact of stress on aging, we hold the key to potentially unlocking a more graceful, attenuated aging process. We're talking about tilting the seesaw of stress and relaxation in your favor, encouraging a sense of balance that allows your body to thrive instead of just survive.

The human body is a marvel of resilience and adaptation. Stress is but one factor in the vast mosaic of aging, and with the right knowledge and tools, its impact can be lessened, allowing you to enjoy a fuller, richer life experience, well into your golden years.

So as you continue to navigate the twisting road of managing aging, keep in the forefront of your mind the substantial role stress plays. Addressing stress isn't just a footnote on the journey to longevity; it's a vital element in ensuring the quality, not just the quantity, of the years you have ahead.

With these insights on stress and its vexing relationship with aging, you're better equipped to tackle the next segment, which promises to guide you through effective stress reduction practices, bringing you closer to that coveted fountain of youthful living, one stress-free step at a time.

Effective Stress Reduction Practices As we move through life, particularly as we age, managing stress becomes not just a luxury, but a necessity. Indeed, mastering the art of stress reduction is tantamount to finding the fountain of youth. It's a silent partner to our longevity, our happiness, and to the graceful aging we all seek. In this section, let's unfold some effective stress reduction practices that are both practical and empowering.

Let's start with mindfulness. Mindfulness, a term that echoes through the corridors of modern stress management approaches, is about being fully present. Engaging in mindfulness exercises—like paying close attention to your breath, or savoring each bite of your meal—can serve as an anchor, pulling you away from the stressors of life and into the tranquility of the moment.

Meditation, often seen as the sister practice to mindfulness, takes the idea deeper. It's about setting aside dedicated time to calm the mind. Whether you choose guided meditations, silent contemplation, or practices like transcendental meditation, the key is consistency. Neuroscience applauds meditation for its ability to literally rewire the brain for peace, and from this peace, a younger, vibrant self can emerge.

Don't overlook the power of deep breathing. When done consciously, deep breathing activates the parasympathetic nervous system, signaling your body to relax. This can be a quick way to de-escalate stress anywhere, anytime. Try breathing in deeply to a count of four, holding for a count of four, then exhaling for a count of six. The extended exhale is the secret sauce to calming the nervous system.

Physical exercise, while discussed in detail in earlier chapters, deserves a mention here for its stress-busting powers. Whether it's yoga, running, or dancing, moving your body can help release pent-up tension, clear your mind, and trigger the release of endorphins, the body's natural mood lifters.

A practice gaining momentum is journaling. Writing down thoughts and feelings can create a space for emotional release. Reflecting on your day, expressing gratitude, or venting frustrations onto paper can be incredibly cathartic and a way to lighten the mental load we often carry.

Laughter, often said to be the best medicine, is a bona fide stress reliever. It releases endorphins and relaxes the whole body. Furthermore, it's thought that laughter may boost the immune system and reduce inflammation, which are crucial in combatting the effects of aging. So, seek out humor in your day-to-day life—whether it's through social connections, movies, or even laughter yoga classes.

Speaking of social connections, building and maintaining social networks can provide emotional support and create a buffer against stress. Sharing your experiences with friends or participating in community activities can create a sense of belonging and self-worth, vital for stress management.

Creative endeavors such as painting, music, or gardening can also act as therapeutic outlets for stress. They focus the mind on the task at hand and away from the cyclical patterns of stressful thoughts. Plus, there's a sense of accomplishment in creating something that adds to the feel-good factor.

A sometimes underestimated tool in the stress relief arsenal is the power of nature. Studies suggest that spending time outdoors, particularly in green spaces, can lower stress levels, improve mood, and even enhance cognitive function. Whether it's a walk in the park, a hike in the woods, or just sitting in the garden, the effects are tangible.

Adequate sleep, which we've explored in previous chapters, cannot be emphasized enough. It's critical for resetting the brain and body. A lack of sleep can lead to an increase in stress hormones, which in turn can exacerbate the aging process. Thus, having a solid nighttime routine and practicing good sleep hygiene plays directly into your stress management and anti-aging strategy.

Let's not forget about healthy eating—when your body is nourished with the right foods, it's better equipped to handle stress. A diet rich in antioxidants, healthy fats, and lean proteins can support the nervous system and lower inflammation, providing a stable foundation to combat stress.

Time management is another practical approach to reducing stress. By learning to prioritize tasks, avoid overcommitment, and delegate when necessary, you can reduce the overwhelm that often accelerates the feeling of frantic aging.

Lastly, it's essential to learn the fine art of saying "no." Setting boundaries is crucial for mental health and stress reduction. By not overextending yourself and protecting your time, you prioritize your well-being, which is a critical component of aging well.

Embrace these stress reduction practices, and you're not just looking at a calmer existence but a potentially extended and more vibrant life. Remember that managing stress isn't about eliminating every challenging situation from your life, but about cultivating resilience and finding peace amid chaos. By integrating these practices into your life, you're paving the way for a long, healthy, and flourishing existence well into your golden years.

Chapter 8:
Skin Care Secrets

Gliding through the preceding chapters, we've armored ourselves with a robust understanding of how the aging process can be maneuvered through diet, fitness, and stress management. Now, let's turn our focus to the canvas that often betrays the very essence of our age—the skin. Truly, skin doesn't lie; it reflects our life's path, illustrating our history and essentially, the passage of time. However, layers upon layers, our epidermal sheath holds secrets, waiting to be unlocked, that can defy those creeping chronological changes. Thriving skin requires more than a casual slather of lotions and serums; it beckons for a regimen, a careful curation of daily practices that honor its complex needs while warding off the relentless march of time. As we delve into the world of ceramides, peptides, and antioxidants, it becomes increasingly clear that what we nourish our bodies with is just as critical as our topical arsenals. The dermal truths unveil themselves through a symbiosis of internal vibrancy and external care, where each day presents an opportunity to imbue our skin with youthful resilience. In this chapter, I'll usher you through those rituals and realities that pave the way to skin that doesn't just aspire to reclaim younger days but radiates a newfound, enduring luminescence.

Daily Routines for Ageless Skin Embracing the notion that our skin is just as dynamic as the rest of our body, it's only natural to focus on nurturing it with the steadfast dedication we give to our overall health. To weave the tapestry of ageless skin, there's a symphony of rituals to conduct daily. We don't just stumble upon radiant skin; we strategize, we dedicate, and we commit to routines as timeless as the results we seek.

Beyond fancy creams and serums, the true secret to ageless skin lies in the daily acts of love we show our outermost selves. In the morning, a gentle cleanser sets the stage—not stripping away, but rather preparing the skin. It's about working *with* your biological masterpiece, not against it. Post-cleansing, we layer our canvases with antioxidants - think vitamin C serums that guard against the environmental onslaught of free radicals.

Finding solace in the shade is as vital as any product we apply. Sun protection is non-negotiable. We're talking broad-spectrum sunscreen, reapplied every two hours, diligently. It's not vanity; it's about defending our skin's integrity from the relentless sun. We adorn hats and seek shade, not out of fear, but out of respect for the power of nature's star.

As we bathe in the glory of the daytime rituals, transitioning to nightfall paves the way for recovery and renewal. We unburden our skin of the day's adventures with the same tender cleanse. But at night, we invite different players onto the field - retinoids, those cell-turnover prodigies, take the stage to support skin regeneration whilst we dive deep into our slumber.

Hydration is the unsung hero. It's not just gulping down water, but integrating moisture rich in hyaluronic acid, and locking it in with effective emollients. We gently pat our faces, distributing creams that replenish what the hours of wakefulness have siphoned away, and with each tap, we're whispering affirmations of health and longevity.

Then there's the diet; our skin feeds on what we eat. A rainbow of vegetables and fruits becomes the best kind of fuel—delivering vitamins, minerals, and antioxidants that our skin craves. Their colors aren't just a treat for the eyes, but a feast for the skin. What we pinch between our forks is as important as what we dab on our cheeks.

Moving along, exercise finds its way into our skincare routine too. Through sweat, we release toxins, and through circulation, we deliver nutrients. It's not about high impact, but being consistent in keeping our bodies—and by extension, our skin—active and oxygenated.

Sleep quality enters as the next piece of the puzzle. As we drift away in the night, our bodies enter repair mode. Redefining "beauty sleep", we view rest not just as a reprieve, but as an essential period where our skin cells replace and heal themselves, unassisted by our conscious efforts, guided only by the sophistication of our biology.

We learn to handle stress with grace—not for the sole sake of mental serenity, but recognizing the tangible cascade it unleashes upon our skin. Stress management is a pillar; with meditative breaths, we not only calm our minds but soothe our skin. Cortisol, the stress hormone, can be as abrasive to our dermal cells as an exfoliant scrub. Gentle is the keyword here, always.

Touch becomes a tool. We employ gentle facial massage techniques to improve lymphatic drainage, to shape and stimulate. It's not rigorous, just gentle upward strokes, encouraging our skin to defy gravity, to retain its spring and vitality through thoughtful, deliberate motion.

We must not underestimate the impact of our surroundings. Clean air, a moderate environment—free from harsh heating or aggressive air conditioning—keeps our skin serene. We opt for humidifiers when necessary, maintaining a balance that mirrors our skin's natural habitat, honoring its preferences as we do our own comfort.

Constantly evolving, our routines adjust to the demands of time and change. We stay keenly attuned to our skin's dialogues, embracing seasonal shifts, hormonal fluctuations, and lifestyle transitions with adjustments in our skincare routine that reflect a dynamic understanding of our body's largest organ.

Beyond individual products or discrete choices, it's the cumulative commitment, the repeated rituals, and consistency that truly hallmark the quest for ageless skin. We can't capture youth in a bottle, but we can cultivate it through daily disciplines, turning routines into rites of passage that honor our journey towards lifelong vitality.

Integrating the wisdom we've garnered from both cutting-edge science and ancestral traditions, we piece together regimens that work not only on our skin's surface but also resonate deeper within. The goal of this chapter is not to prescribe a universal elixir but to cultivate a mindset. Ageless skin is not just skin that looks youthful—it's skin cared for with foresight, intention and the reverence it deserves in the narrative of our lives.

Together, these daily habits form a mosaic of care that, over time, results in a complexion that doesn't betray the passing of years but celebrates the wisdom they bring. As the layers of our skin renew, so does our commitment to the practices that replenish and protect them. This dialogue between us and our skin, through routines basked in care, becomes the alchemy through which the ageless quality we seek is not just envisioned but embodied.

The Truth About Anti-Aging Products In the world of skin care, the siren song of anti-aging products is alluring—it promises the fountain of youth in a bottle. Walk into any cosmetics aisle and you're bombarded with an array of creams, serums and lotions touting miraculous results. But the truth? Not all that glitters is gold.

Peering beyond the shiny façades and brushed metal packages, what's actually lurking inside these concoctions can be a bit of a mixed bag. To be clear, there are products out there that certainly have the potential to improve skin health and appearance. But, and it's a big but, it's vital to approach them with a discerning eye, fully understanding their limitations and benefits.

The science of skincare has made incredible strides, especially concerning ingredients like retinoids, peptides, hyaluronic acid, and various antioxidants. These ingredients have shown promise in reducing the appearance of wrinkles, fine lines, and other visual hallmarks of aging. They work by encouraging the skin to behave more youthfully—boosting collagen production, enhancing cellular turnover, and fighting oxidative stress.

Yet, it's critical to manage expectations. While some ingredients have earned their accolade in peer-reviewed studies, the results aren't always as dramatic as advertised. Anti-aging products might improve skin texture and tone, but they can't reverse time. They can't change your genetic makeup, and they can't completely eradicate the effects of years of sun exposure, pollution, diet, and personal habits.

Moreover, the concentration of these active ingredients matters. An over-the-counter product might contain a much lower concentration of a scientifically-backed component than what was used in clinical studies, leading to less significant results. It's much like getting a diluted version of a potent elixir; you're not quite getting the punch the studies are talking about.

When considering anti-aging products, the integrity and formulation of a product are just as important as the active ingredients. A well-formulated product will have a stable shelf life, maintain the integrity of its active ingredients, and be able to deliver those ingredients effectively to the skin. On the other hand, a poorly formulated product, no matter how good the ingredients list looks, can do more harm than good.

Caveat emptor—buyer beware. While some products deliver on some of their promises, others may be filled with nothing more than empty promises and exotic-sounding ingredients designed to captivate your imagination rather than deliver results. It's vital to scrutinize ingredients, understand what they do, and verify whether there's solid science backing their efficacy.

And then there's the question of cost. High price tags often accompany anti-aging skincare products, but a hefty price doesn't always equate to effectiveness. Some inexpensive products contain similar concentrations of key ingredients as their luxury counterparts. It pays to do your research and understand whether you're paying for results or just the brand perception and marketing.

It is essential to prioritize overall skin health over the pursuit of anti-aging promises. A well-rounded skincare routine that includes sun protection, moisturization, and gentle cleansing can go a long way toward maintaining skin's appearance and health. Healthy skin will naturally look more youthful, regardless of the number of anti-aging products in your cabinet.

Let's not overlook the place of lifestyle in the fight against aging. No serum can outmatch the profound effects of a balanced diet, regular exercise, adequate sleep, and stress management. In essence, those looking for a single miraculous solution are often missing out on the holistic approach required for real, substantive results.

As we explore anti-aging products, we should keep an open mind to the potential benefits of incremental improvements. Small gains in skin hydration or elasticity may not sound like headline news, but over time, these benefits accumulate, contributing to a complexion that can resist some of the common signs of aging.

This speaks to the wisdom of long-term investment in skin health rather than quick fixes. A regimen that incorporates products with well-supported ingredients, used consistently and complemented by a healthy lifestyle, could create the foundation for a genuinely age-defying complexion.

Lastly, think of skin care as a personal journey rather than a universal solution. Everyone's skin is different; what works wonders for one person may not be as effective for another. It's important to tailor your skincare routine to your unique needs and responses, possibly with the help of a dermatologist.

Anti-aging products can certainly play a role in an overall strategy for maintaining refined and vibrant skin. But they're only a part of the equation. They're not the panacea, but a tool—one of many—for those striving to manage the visible signs of aging. It's this blend of insight, realistic expectations, and persistent care that sets the stage for skin that ages gracefully, reflecting the vivacity and resilience of the person within.

Chapter 9:
Hormonal Balance and Aging

The delicate dance of hormones within our bodies is a performance that doesn't always get the standing ovation it deserves, yet it's pivotal to our journey through aging. We've peeked beneath the skin to unveil the mysteries of cellular clocks and explored the terrain of nutritional goldmines, but let's pivot to an oft-overlooked realm: the endocrine system. As we age, it's no secret that the body's production of certain hormones shifts, sometimes subtly, sometimes with a more pronounced impact. This chapter dives into the natural lifelines of hormonal balance, spearheading the vanishing act of age marks and energy dips. It's like having a backstage pass to the endocrine system, offering privileged insights on how to coax hormones into a harmonious chorus that supports vitality, rather than heralding decline. Strategies for natural hormone balance aren't one-size-fits-all, of course; they require a tailored approach that listens to the body's cues with attentive care. You'll find that with the right lifestyle choices, from sleep patterns to stress management, you can conduct the hormonal symphony in a way that breathes life into every cell and keeps that biological clock ticking with precision and grace.

The Endocrine System's Role in Aging Stepping inland from the chapters that sculpt our approach to aging, we come across a pivotal player in the grand performance of our lives—the endocrine system. This complex network of glands and hormones is the maestro that conducts the symphony of our bodily functions, and as we age, it's this very conductor that could start missing a beat here and there.

Hormones are the body's chemical messengers, and the endocrine system, which produces these hormones, plays a crucial role in maintaining health and vitality. This system adjusts and calibrates essential processes such as metabolism, growth, sleep, and reproduction. As we step into the later chapters of life, our bodily processes, guided by the endocrine system, naturally shift, signaling the body to enter a new phase.

Think of the thyroid gland, a workhorse that regulates metabolism, energy, and even our mood. As we age, it's common for thyroid function to dwindle, often leading to hypothyroidism—where our metabolic processes slow down, resulting in fatigue, weight gain, and a decline in cognitive functions.

And let's not skirt around the topic of the 'change of life', or menopause in women and andropause in men. These are natural life stages with a cocktail of hormonal changes, predominantly in the sex hormones—estrogen, progesterone, and testosterone. The consequences? They range from hot flashes and mood swings to a more profound risk of osteoporosis and heart disease.

We see the adrenals, those tiny hats that sit atop the kidneys, pumping out cortisol in response to stress. In youth, they adeptly manage stress levels, but over time, too much cortisol can be churning out, or too little when it's most needed, making our response to stress less than ideal. This can increase the risk of chronic diseases and impact our ability to recover from everyday stressors.

Now, behold the pancreas—an organ with a firm handshake between the endocrine and digestive systems. It secretes insulin, a hormone that helps regulate blood sugar levels. With age, cells can become more resistant to insulin's effects, a condition known as insulin resistance, inching us closer to type 2 diabetes—a significant public health concern impacting aging populations worldwide.

Granted, it's hard not to notice the influence of the pituitary gland, sometimes called the 'master gland', as it orchestrates the production of many other hormones within the body. With time's passage, changes in its function can affect a multitude of systems, showing that even the master isn't immune to the effects of aging.

Yet, amid these inevitable changes, there's good news. Lifestyle choices play a monumental role in how our bodies cope with the hormonal shifts due to aging. Engaging in regular physical activity is akin to serenading our endocrine system, encouraging a fine balance among our hormone levels. Exercise alone can boost metabolism, improve insulin sensitivity, and build muscle mass, offsetting some of the signs of hormonal aging.

Our diet, rich in nutrients and low in processed foods, influences our endocrine health too. Foods that stabilize blood sugar and provide adequate amounts of vitamins and minerals can bolster our glands in their aging battles. Similarly, adequate sleep and stress reduction techniques are the balm that soothes a weary endocrine system, helping to maintain hormonal harmony well into the twilight years.

Further to this, the growing field of bioidentical hormone replacement therapy offers nuanced approaches to replenish hormones that have declined with age. While this should be navigated with careful medical supervision, it represents a frontier in managing aging, often bringing renewed vigor to those who tread its path.

Looking to the horizon, advancements in anti-aging medicine and personalized medicine are promising beacons. They're creating innovative ways to support the endocrine system, tapping into genetic insights and tailoring interventions that keep our hormone cascades flowing gracefully.

Proactive monitoring is also vital as aging veers closer. Routine medical check-ups, including hormone level evaluations, can catch early signs of endocrine imbalance, allowing for timely interventions. This highlights the importance of understanding our bodies and advocating for our health as we age.

Yet, while medicine continues to evolve, the simple universal truth remains: balance is the golden key. A balanced approach to living—a synergy of nutrition, exercise, sleep, and emotional well-being—can be our best strategy against the tide of time that interacts so intimately with our endocrine system.

As we navigate the following chapters that delve deeper into specifics, let's hold onto the thought that aging is not merely a decline but a new stage with its potential for growth. Our body's incredible endocrine orchestra does not have to play a somber tune if we learn how to conduct it with attentiveness and care. There's beauty in this biological complexity, and with the right notes, we can transform this part of our life into a harmonious melody.

So, as we continue our pursuit of longevity, let's listen to the whispers of our endocrine system and respond with choices that align with its needs. After all, the dance with our hormones is one of the most poignant in the ballet of aging—it's about learning the steps to aging gracefully and, in doing so, finding the rhythm of a life well-lived.

Natural Ways to Maintain Hormonal Health As we move through this vibrant tapestry that is the journey of aging, we've touched on the myriad facets that contribute to our well-being. We've navigated through the pivotal role of diet, the transformative power of physical activity, and the soothing embrace of proper sleep. Yet, amidst this mosaic of health, the subtle and profound influence of hormones often goes understated. Hormones are the body's chemical messengers, orchestrating a symphony of biological processes that maintain balance and vitality as we age.

One natural avenue for sustaining hormonal health is through the foods we eat. Cruciferous vegetables, like broccoli and cauliflower, are not just culinary delights; they are also warriors in balancing hormones, particularly estrogen. They contain compounds such as indole-3-carbinol, which helps in modulating estrogen and potentially reducing the risk of hormone-related cancers.

Another cornerstone of hormonal harmony is the consumption of healthy fats. Our endocrine system relies on these fats for the construction of hormones. Avocados, olive oil, and nuts are rich in monounsaturated fats, while fatty fish like salmon brim with omega-3 fatty acids. These foods don't just satiate our palates; they fortify our hormonal resilience against the tides of time.

Let's not underestimate the potency of physical activity in this narrative. Regular exercise doesn't just sculpt the physique or bolster the heart; it also primes our hormones. When we engage in movement, our bodies release endorphins, the feel-good hormones, which in turn can regulate stress hormones like cortisol. This balancing act is instrumental in mitigating the stress-related accelerators of aging.

Moreover, the art of mindfulness, deeply rooted in the practice of controlling breath and intention, can manifest as a powerful conductor of hormonal balance. Practices like yoga and tai chi, which integrate mindful breathing, have been shown to reduce stress hormones and promote relaxation, fostering an internal environment where hormones can flourish.

Stepping into the realm of sleep, we find yet another ally for hormonal health. A well-rested body is a fertile ground for proper hormonal function. Consistent, quality sleep supports the regulation of growth hormone, which plays an invaluable role in tissue repair and muscle maintenance—an essential consideration as we age.

Herbal adaptogens, like ashwagandha and rhodiola, have long been heralded in traditional medicine systems for their hormone-modulating effects. These herbs are believed to bolster our body's resilience to stress and aids in balancing stress hormones, indirectly supporting overall hormonal health.

Hydration, often oversimplified as mere thirst-quenching, serves as a lynchpin in hormonal balance. Adequate water intake ensures that the blood can transport hormones to their destined sites of action effectively. The simple act of drinking enough water each day is akin to keeping the lines of communication open and clear within our body.

Then there's the necessity of maintaining a healthy body weight. Excessive adipose tissue, or body fat, can throw a wrench in the works when it comes to hormone levels, notably insulin and estrogen. A balanced diet, paired with regular physical activity, can aid in managing weight and thus, hormonal equilibrium.

Moving on, we look to the diverse food groups that supply a medley of nutrients essential for hormone production. For instance, pumpkin seeds, rich in zinc, are crucial for testosterone production, while vitamin D, abundantly found in fortified foods and sunlight, is central to the synthesis of several hormones. These nutrients are the building blocks that support our endocrine system as we age.

Environmental toxins and endocrine disruptors, found in plastics and pesticides, can be silent saboteurs of our hormonal health. By opting for organic produce and reducing plastic usage, we can mitigate exposure to these disruptors, curating a cleaner slate for our hormones to operate on.

Stress management is paramount, as chronic stress can wreak havoc on our endocrine system, with cortisol being a prime instigator.

Techniques like deep breathing, progressive muscle relaxation, and guided imagery can restore a sense of calm and rebalance our hormonal scales.

Don't overlook the importance of social connections; engaging in heartwarming interactions with friends and family can release oxytocin, often dubbed the 'love hormone,' which plays a pivotal role in fostering bonding and reducing stress levels.

Lastly, the role of periodic fasting or time-restricted eating in hormonal health cannot be ignored. Intermittent fasting can improve insulin sensitivity, regulate ghrelin and leptin, the hunger and satiety hormones, and stimulate autophagy, a cellular clean-up process that may impact hormone receptors' longevity and sensitivity.

Every piece of this puzzle, from what rests on our forks to the tranquility of our minds, from the environment in which we live to the activities that invigorate our beings, coalesces into a comprehensive approach to natural hormonal health.

As you journey through these pages, let each chapter not merely be words on a page but stepping stones towards an empowered existence. Embracing these natural strategies for maintaining hormonal health is not just a whim of the health-conscious—it's an integral part of the symphony that will allow us to dance gracefully with time, ensuring our later years glimmer with vitality.

Chapter 10:
Brain Health and Cognitive Function

As we've explored the body's physical rejuvenation, we now turn our focus to the unfathomable complexity of the human brain. In the realm of long-term wellbeing, maintaining cognitive sharpness is just as crucial as a steady heartbeat or a glowing complexion. It's your brain's orchestration of neurons and synapses that enables you to savor memories, solve puzzles, and connect with loved ones. So, what's the secret to safeguarding these priceless treasures against the wear of time? It's not just about crossword puzzles or the occasional Sudoku—though they have their place. Instead, think of brain health as a lush, vibrant garden that requires diverse seeds of nutrition, exercise, and mental challenges to flourish. Within this chapter, we will unearth the layers of cognitive care, shedding light on how specific nutrients can serve as your neural knights in shining armor, and unveiling exercises that not only tone muscles but also sharpen the mind. This isn't just about avoiding decline; it's a proactive quest to elevate your mental acuity to new heights, ensuring that your cognitive garden blossoms, resilient and thriving, throughout the tapestry of your years.

Exercises to Keep Your Mind Sharp As we've journeyed through the myriad avenues to preserve youth and navigate the aging process, we've now arrived at the crux of sustaining cognitive vitality. Like the muscles in our body that require regular training to maintain tone and function, our brain, an often-overlooked organ in fitness, demands a workout regimen all its own to remain sharp and agile.

Let's begin with something we all enjoy, puzzles. Crossword puzzles, Sudoku, and brainteasers aren't merely pastimes; they are cognitive calisthenics that fortify your brain's prowess. They compel you to think critically, solve problems creatively, and focus with unwavering attention. Integrating these into your routine can transform idle moments into opportunities for mental fortification.

Next up is the power of memory exercises. Commit to learning something new daily, whether it's a fact, a poem, or a series of numbers. Challenge yourself to recall it later, engaging your memory muscles and enhancing recall abilities. It could be as simple as remembering the names of new acquaintances or as complex as memorizing a new language's vocabulary.

Musical instruments aren't just for the musically inclined; they're for anyone seeking to sharpen their mind. Learning to play an instrument later in life can significantly improve hand-eye coordination, listening skills, and memory recall. The intricacies of music theory also promote complex thought processes and problem-solving skills, offering cognitive benefits akin to learning a new language.

Speaking of languages, becoming bilingual or multilingual is a powerful neuroprotective activity. Language learning stimulates new neural pathways, improves problem-solving, and can even delay the onset of dementia. It's like a gym session for your brain with a lifetime membership of benefits.

Regular reading is fundamental—no pun intended—for keeping your mind supple. Delving into books stimulates imagination, expands vocabulary, and increases knowledge. Moreover, the focus and concentration required during reading is like a meditation session for your cognitive functions, calming the mind while simultaneously sharpening it.

Writing, whether creative storytelling or journaling your thoughts, is an excellent tool for mental clarity. It encourages you to think deeply, articulate your ideas clearly, and enhance language skills. Writing by hand, in particular, can also improve neural activity and memory recall.

Board games and strategy games aren't just for kids or game nights; they're essential tools for adults to maintain strategic thinking and foresight. Games like chess, Scrabble, or even modern video games require complex thought and strategy, which help to keep the brain engaged and nimble.

Physical exercise should not be discounted when considering mental acuity. Activities like yoga, tai chi, or even brisk walking increase blood flow to the brain, delivering oxygen and vital nutrients. What benefits the heart, benefits the brain—it's all interconnected.

Lifelong learning is not just an idealistic phrase; it's a practical approach to keeping your intellect razor-sharp. Take up courses in subjects you're unfamiliar with, attend lectures, or watch educational documentaries. The key is to consistently introduce your brain to new concepts and challenges.

Let's not forget the simple act of socialization. Engaging in thoughtful conversations, debates, or social activities stimulate your mind. The dynamic nature of human interaction forces your brain to adapt, understand different perspectives, and process information on the fly, providing a robust mental workout.

Meditation, though often associated with emotional and spiritual wellbeing, also plays a substantial role in brain health. Even a few minutes a day has shown to improve focus, reduce stress—which, as we know impairs cognitive function—and even boost gray matter in the brain.

Visualization and mind-mapping techniques can be powerful tools for brain health. They help in organizing thoughts, planning projects, or even visualizing success, which stimulates strategic thinking and memory.

And what of cooking? Surprising as it may be, cooking activates various cognitive processes including, attention, planning, and multi-tasking. Following new recipes enhances comprehension and execution functions, while the sensory experiences improve recognition and recall.

Moving into more immersive experiences, virtual reality (VR) has shown promise as a cognitive training tool. It offers simulations that can improve spatial awareness, reaction time, and enhance memory through interactive and engaging platforms.

Lastly, never underestimate the value of curiosity. Approaching life with an inquisitive mindset, asking questions, seeking answers, and exploring your world is perhaps the most natural and profound exercise for the mind. It is curiosity that fuels all the other activities we've discussed, and it keeps the mind eternally youthful.

In our pursuit of longevity, we invest ample time in physical health, often sidelining the very organ that orchestrates our every move and thought—the brain. Engaging in exercises that promote cognitive health isn't just about extending lifespan; it's about enriching the quality of every year we gain. So as we continue to learn and adapt across the chapters of our lives, integrating these brain-boosting activities will not only craft a sharper mind but pave the way for a deeper, more vibrant existence as the years progress.

Nutrients That Boost Brain Power As we navigate the topic of brain health and cognitive function, it becomes evident that what we consume can be as significant as a challenging crossword puzzle for keeping our wits sharp. Now, let's delve into the specific nutrients that our cerebral command centers crave for optimal performance. It's not just about dodging forgetfulness or fog; it's about fuelling the mastermind within us for a vibrant, longer life.

Omega-3 fatty acids stand out as true brain-boosting superstars. Found abundantly in fish such as salmon and sardines, these fats are not just builders of cell membranes in the brain but also guardians against cognitive decline. Incorporating omega-3s into your diet can support learning processes and memory retention - it's like an investment in your mental bank account for future years.

Antioxidants also form a protective entourage for your neurons. Vitamin E is particularly adept at this, warding off the damage from free radicals that can lead to brain cell deterioration over time. Almonds, spinach, and sweet potatoes are just a few of the treasure troves for this nutrient. Picture it as armor for your gray matter; a way to combat the rust that the years can bring.

Complex carbohydrates deserve a spot at the table of brain-enhancing nutrients too. These aren't your run-of-the-mill carbs, but fibrous, whole grains that break down slowly and provide a steady stream of glucose - the brain's preferred energy source. Include brown rice or quinoa in your meal and visualize fueling your mental engine for the long-haul.

Let's talk about B vitamins. Emerging as a dynamic team, vitamins B6, B12, and folic acid help reduce levels of homocysteine in the blood, an amino acid linked to cognitive impairment. Think of B vitamins as the cleanup crew that keeps the bloodstream clear for optimal mental function. Legumes, leafy greens, and fortified cereals are great ways to get these nutrients.

Choline, often underappreciated, is another brain booster. A key ingredient in the neurotransmitter acetylcholine, it plays a pivotal role in regulating memory and muscle control. It's as if choline is the communications officer in the brain, making sure messages are sent and received loud and clear. Eggs and soybeans are choline champions, ready to amplify your cognitive clarity.

Are you getting enough iron? It's essential for preventing brain fog, as iron assists in oxygen transport in the blood and plays a crucial role in cognitive development and function. Lack of iron can lead to fatigue and affect concentration. Think of iron-rich foods like lentils and spinach as your personal mental sharpeners, ready to boost your focus.

Zinc is another mineral that's vital for neurological function and mood regulation. It aids neurogenesis, the birth of new neuronal cells, and synaptic plasticity, which is crucial for learning and memory. Pumpkin seeds are a tasty source of this nutrient—just another way to plant the seeds for a sharper mind.

Don't underestimate the importance of water. Hydration is essential for the brain, which is composed of about 75% water. Dehydration can impair attention and short-term memory. Imagine each sip as a way to maintain the supple, fluid nature of your brain tissue, necessary for it to function at its prime.

Caffeine, in moderation, can be a helpful cognitive stimulant, improving reaction times and warding off drowsiness. Yes, that morning cup of coffee might indeed be giving your brain a gentle nudge into wakefulness. Picture caffeine as the spark that lights the flame of alertness, warming up your mental processes for the day ahead.

Protein, packed with amino acids, serves as the building block for neurotransmitters, the brain's chemical messengers. Consuming high-quality proteins from sources such as lean meats, nuts, and tofu, can have a direct impact on cognitive health and performance. View these proteins as the couriers in your brain's postal service, delivering thoughts and commands efficiently and effectively.

Lutein, a carotenoid found in kale and spinach, seems to accumulate in the brain and is believed to play a neuroprotective role. It's like having a personal bodyguard for your neurons, ensuring they do their job without interference from oxidative stress.

Flavonoids, which give berries and dark chocolate their rich coloring, have been associated with better brain function and slower decline in memory. These compounds are the brain's berry-own task force, targeting cognitive functions to renew and protect.

Magnesium is involved in more than 300 biochemical reactions in the body, including neurotransmission and neural excitability. Nuts, seeds, and whole grains are rich in this nutrient, each serving as a cog in the grand machinery of your cognitive processes.

So, what does all this mean for you, the savvy navigator of aging? It means that brain power isn't static; it's dynamic, fueled by the choices you make at mealtime. By ensuring a varied diet rich in the nutrients laid out on this cerebral spread, you're not just eating for today; you're dining for the future of your mental faculties.

Last but certainly not least, let's remember that these nutrients don't work in isolation. They're part of a symphony, each playing its part in a well-rounded diet that supports all aspects of your well-being. Think harmony, think complexity, think diversity—embrace the symphony of nutrition for your brain, and let it play a beautiful melody of cognitive resilience as you age with grace.

Chapter 11:
The Power of Social Connections

As we continue to journey through the myriad ways to bolster our longevity, we find ourselves at the heart of a less tangible, yet incredibly potent facet of well-being: our social ties. In this chapter, we're diving into the profound impact that community and connection have on our health, particularly as we age. Studies have unveiled that cultivating rich social networks isn't just a boon for emotional fulfillment; it's intricately linked to physical health, cognitive function, and even the resilience one has in the face of life's adversities. Think of your friendships and family ties not as just life's accessories, but as lifelines—cords that can anchor us amidst the stormy seas of aging. By actively engaging in our communities, nurturing deep relationships, and valuing quality over quantity in our social interactions, we unlock a treasure trove of anti-aging magic. It's through shared experiences, meaningful conversations, and the simple yet powerful act of belonging that we find a crucial key to unlocking a life that doesn't just span years, but is rich with quality and vitality as well.

Social Engagement and Its Effects on Longevity As we flip the page from understanding individual health pursuits, let's wade into the waters of social engagement. It's a fascinating area that, believe it or not, has a profound impact on how long we might grace this planet. When considering the tapestry of longevity, one of the most vibrant threads is our connection with other people. It's not just about the occasional meet-up or holiday gathering; it's the depth, regularity, and quality of our social interactions that truly make the difference.

It's been shown time and again that humans are inherently social creatures. From the cradle to the cane, the bonds we forge serve as both a comfort blanket and a shield against the proverbial slings and arrows of life. The support systems we create and maintain throughout our lives can determine not only the quality of our days but also their quantity. It almost sounds too good to be true, but science backs it up—social engagement can lead to a longer life.

Think about it; loneliness isn't just a feeling. It's a stressor, and when it becomes chronic, it can wear away at our health like waves against a cliff. It's often linked with higher blood pressure, increased inflammation, and a weakened immune system. Fight or flight responses become overactive when we feel socially isolated, and this can speed up the aging process. Engaging meaningfully with others seems to act like a balm, soothing our stress responses and helping to sustain our well-being.

The benefits aren't just physical; they're psychological too. Our state of mind plays a key role in how we age. Social interaction, from casual chats to deep heart-to-hearts, fuels our sense of belonging and purpose. When people feel valued and connected, it's like a natural vaccine against the despair that sometimes accompanies aging. Moreover, these interactions keep our brains engaged and challenged—vital for cognitive health as the years roll on.

Furthermore, peer pressure isn't always a bad thing. Your social circles can influence your health behaviors, nudging you toward or away from habits that impact your longevity. Surround yourself with friends who prefer walking in the park over an afternoon nap; you'll likely find the energy to lace up your sneakers too. Similarly, if your companions enjoy a diet rich in fruits, veggies, and other whole foods, you're more apt to join the feast—and reap the nutritive rewards.

Volunteering also throws a spotlight on the importance of being socially active. It's a double win; you contribute to society while padding your own health. Being altruistic through volunteer work enhances your self-esteem, decreases depressive symptoms, and can even lead to reduced mortality rates. That warm glow you get from helping others? It's your body saying 'thank you' for engaging with the world in a meaningful way.

That's not to say you need a rolodex full of contacts to live a long, fulfilling life. The key is in the quality of connections rather than the quantity. A few close, supportive relationships can be just as beneficial as a wide social network. Deeply connecting with family, friends, or even pets can create an emotional buffer against the stressors that age us.

As we get older, maintaining these connections can become more challenging. Life throws curveballs—friends move away, loved ones pass on, and we retire from work environments that once provided daily interaction. It's vital to adapt and find new ways to engage. Senior centers, community classes, online forums—these can be the bridges to new relationships and maintained engagement. They provide avenues for laughter, learning, and love, crucial ingredients for a long and happy life.

There's also a hint of reciprocity in the relationship between social engagement and longevity. It's not just that being social keeps you living longer; living longer encourages you to maintain social connections. Picture it as a cycle where one good turn leads to another, and your investment in relationships pays dividends in added years.

Lest we ignore those who enjoy solitude, it's essential to balance alone time with social activity. Solitude can be replenishing, a chance to reflect and recharge. But too much alone time might risk tipping the scales towards isolation. Striking a balance is crucial.

Staying socially active doesn't require grand gestures. Sometimes, it's the small, consistent acts—weekly phone calls to a friend, joining a book club, attending a local event—that keep the social wheel turning. Staying engaged means staying interested in others and the world around you, learning new things, sharing experiences, and creating memories.

And for the younger generations, it's a worthwhile endeavor to not just focus on building careers and individual achievements, but also to cultivate strong, supportive social circles. Starting this practice early paves the way for a rich web of relationships that sustains you through life's ebbs and flows.

So, there we have it—the science is clear, and the anecdotes affirm: Social engagement is a pillar upon which the temple of longevity is built. As you move forward in the journey of life, remember that the hands you hold, the conversations you treasure, and the lives you touch may just be the secret to your own vibrant, extended existence.

By emphasizing social connectivity, we are nurturing a fundamental aspect of our health that, too often, is left to the wayside. It's crucial to recognize that social engagement is indispensable, not just for a good life, but for a long one. So reach out, connect, and revel in the community you create—it's one of the most life-affirming choices you can make.

As we explore further aspects of well-being in the subsequent chapters, these principles of social engagement will weave their way into discussions about community and relationships. They will echo in the conversations about brain health, hormonal balance, and the myriad components that construct our intricate mosaic of aging well.

In the next section, we'll delve into the fine art of building and maintaining these healthy relationships. It's one thing to understand the value of connections; it's another altogether to foster and keep them. Grab your social toolkit; we're about to add some new instruments.

Building and Maintaining Healthy Relationships As we navigate through the undulating path of aging, the tapestry of our lives is bolstered by the intricate threads of relationships we maintain. Let's delve deeper into why these connections are not just the icing on the cake, but vital ingredients that help maintain a youthful essence, both emotionally and mentally, as we progress through the years.

The fabric of our social lives comprises of a multitude of relationships: friendships, family ties, romantic partnerships, and professional connections. These bonds shape our experiences, influence our happiness, and can impact our longevity in surprising ways. In fact, studies have indicated that strong relationships may be just as critical to our well-being as avoiding cigarettes and excess alcohol. Now, isn't that something to ponder?

So, what does it take to build and nurture these valuable connections? It starts with communication. Engaging in meaningful conversations, actively listening, and expressing ourselves with clarity fortifies the foundation of any relationship. It's about more than just verbal exchanges; it's about ensuring that you're comprehensible and receptive.

Trust is the cornerstone of any healthy relationship. It's built over time, through consistent and reliable behavior. Trust isn't simply about believing that someone will not betray you; it's also about feeling confident that they will be there for you, providing a stable base of security and support.

Empathy is another crucial component. Stepping into someone else's shoes and viewing the world from their perspective enriches your understanding and patience. Empathy builds bridges and breaks down walls, allowing for deeper connections that endure the test of time.

We can't talk about healthy relationships without mentioning boundaries. Knowing where you end and someone else begins is essential for mutual respect and personal well-being. Boundaries are the personal policies that guide how we engage with others, ensuring our relationships are reciprocal and satisfying.

Also, remember that relationships are not static; they're dynamic and require regular nurturing to thrive. This could mean scheduling regular check-ins with friends or setting up date nights with a partner. It's about making conscious efforts to remain connected and involved in each other's lives, rather than letting valuable relationships dwindle due to neglect.

As we age, the quality of our relationships often takes precedence over quantity. It becomes more about who you can rely on for a hearty laugh, a shoulder to cry on, or wise counsel. Cultivating these quality relationships often requires us to be discerning about whom we invest our time and energy in.

What about when conflicts arise? Arguably, handling disagreements with wisdom is an art form in itself. It's about finding common ground and compromise while being open to change and growth. These moments, when managed well, can strengthen bonds rather than weaken them.

It's also essential to diversify your social portfolio. Just as financial advisers recommend a varied investment portfolio, having a mix of relationships across different ages, backgrounds, and perspectives can enrich your life and provide a robust support system.

Some fear that technology is eroding our social skills, but let's flip the script. Use it to your advantage! In this digital age, staying connected—even across vast distances—is a click away. Video calls, social media, and instant messaging have all made it easier to keep in touch. However, it's still critical to maintain a balance and not let virtual interactions wholly replace the irreplaceable warmth of face-to-face communication.

Volunteering and community involvement present another avenue for fostering relationships. Joining a group or a cause you're passionate about can connect you with others who share your values and interests. These activities not only bolster your social network but also provide a sense of purpose and fulfillment.

For older adults, especially, maintaining social activities can be instrumental in keeping them mentally and physically agile. Retirement brings more free time, which can be filled with social pursuits that maintain cognitive functioning and keep the spirit youthful.

Let's not forget the relationship we have with ourselves. Self-love and self-care are not about ego or narcissism; they're about acknowledging your worth and giving yourself the same kindness you would extend to a dear friend. This internal relationship sets the tone for how you engage with others and accept love and care in return.

Lastly, remember that saying goodbye to certain relationships can also be a part of maintaining overall health. As we discern what serves us best, we may find that letting go of certain ties is necessary. Doing so respectfully and honestly can free up emotional space for more rewarding connections.

In the dance of life, as we twirl and step through the years, maintaining the rhythm of connectivity is key to our happiness and health. The relationships we build and care for are the silent whispers that keep our inner youth alive, echoing the laughs shared, the tears wiped, and the hands held. These connections, invisible yet strong, give us sustenance, adding both years to our life and life to our years.

Chapter 12:
The Role of Supplements

Navigating from the intimately social aspects of aging, let's pivot to a topic with a more tangible bent—the role that supplements can play in our age-defying arsenal. It's a market flooded with promises of youth and vigor, but what's the real scoop? Well, amid the maze of multivitamins, omega-3s, and antioxidants, there lies a kernel of truth to the notion that certain supplements can indeed support the aging process with grace. Now, we're not suggesting that there's a magic pill capable of turning back the hands of time, but rather that a smart, informed approach to supplementation can fill the nutritional potholes left by our modern diets. In this chapter, we'll sift through the evidence, balancing potential benefits against the science, to discern which nutrients might be worthy allies in our quest for longevity. We'll explore which vitamins and minerals have shown real promise and how herbal supplements could play a supportive, albeit sometimes complex, role. This isn't about chasing after an elixir of life but rather making judicious, strategic choices to enhance our well-being as we accumulate those cherished years.

Vitamins and Minerals for Anti-Aging As we foray deeper into the realms of nurturing our bodies for longevity, we land squarely in the midst of an essential conversation: the role of vitamins and minerals in anti-aging. These microscopic marvels are more than just footnotes on a nutrition label; they are vital co-conspirators in our quest to remain youthful and vibrant.

The skin, our most tangible marker of age, hungers for vitamin A. This vitamin doesn't just wage a knightly fight against wrinkles; it staunchly defends against the dullness and dryness that can betray our years. A worthy ally indeed, vitamin A, in the form of retinol creams, has been shown to stimulate collagen production – that springy scaffold beneath our skin that keeps it plump and youthful.

Let's not forget the sunshine vitamin – vitamin D. While basking in the sun's glow can feel rejuvenating, it's the boost in vitamin D synthesis that truly helps our bodies remain lithe and strong. This vitamin fortifies bones, potentially warding off osteoporosis, an unwelcome herald of advanced years. And yet, the plot thickens as studies suggest a robust vitamin D level is linked to a decreased risk of chronic diseases, many of which accelerate aging.

Vitamin E emerges as a dexterous defender in our anti-aging arsenal. Its antioxidant properties bat away harmful free radicals, environmental culprits that can fast-track aging. But there's a subtler art that vitamin E plays: maintaining skin hydration and integrity, fostering a complexion that beams with the gloss of youth.

C-Victory – not a war chant but a term I have coined for the triumphs of vitamin C in our ceaseless battle against the clock. It is, after all, a potent antioxidant that aids in the repair and regeneration of tissues, on top of being a foundational pillar in collagen production. This is the rejuvenation warrior whose daily intake we dare not neglect, for it guards both dermal and internal vitality.

Then there's the B-vitamin brigade, tirelessly keeping our metabolic processes running smoothly. Of particular note is niacin (vitamin B3), which besides being a crucial player in energy production, is gaining respect for its repertoire in skin care – it soothes, moisturizes, and reduces the appearance of fine lines. Folate (vitamin B9) supports cell division and renewal, while biotin (vitamin B7) maintains lush hair and sturdy nails, signals of health and youth that we often take for granted.

Our attention turns now to the mineral magistrates - starting with zinc. This trace element doesn't just bolster the immune system; it also plays a part in cell division and growth. It's a behind-the-scenes artisan in preserving skin's robustness, acting much like a diligent custodian repairing wear and tear.

Magnesium, the master mineral, orchestrates an ensemble of biological symphonies that sing to the tune of youth. It aids in over three hundred enzyme reactions and is elemental for heart health. Its deficiency can manifest in unwelcome ways, from muscle weakness to a diminished zest for life. Equilibrium in magnesium levels, therefore, is a sewn-in seam in the tapestry of aging well.

Calcium, the stalwart gatekeeper of bone density, is a celebrity for good reason. As we age, maintaining a skeletal framework resistant to the brittleness of time is of paramount importance. Calcium's fame is well-deserved; it plays a leading role in keeping our internal architecture sturdy and resilient.

Iron plays an essential yet delicate role in our vitality. It's the core component of hemoglobin, the oxygen-transporting virtuoso in our blood. Ensuring adequate iron levels, especially in postmenopausal women, ushers a flow of oxygen that nurtures organs and keeps lethargy at bay.

Selenium, though less spoken of, deserves its turn in the spotlight. With prowess in preserving elasticity of tissues, this mineral is integral to a supple, graceful aging process. It also assists the body in quelling inflammation, often an insidious accomplice in the deterioration associated with growing old.

Let us wade into the waters of Omega-3 fatty acids, which, though not vitamins or minerals perse, rise to such prominence in anti-aging discussions that they warrant a courteous mention. They are, after all, the lubricants that keep our cell membranes supple, our joints dancing, and our cognition as sharp as the morning horizon.

Embrace the mantra 'balance and moderation', for these vitamins and minerals work not in isolation, but in concert. Now imagine orchestrating this symphony with harmony and precision. Too little, and like an unfinished symphony, we may not reach our full potential. Too much, and the melody may become cacophonous, disrupting other bodily processes.

And as we turn our gaze towards whole foods that are naturally rife with these nutrients, let's remember that every colorful vegetable, every piece of succulent fruit, and every handful of nuts and seeds are tiny packets of anti-aging prowess. Supplements, too, can play a role, but conscious, dietary choices pave the surest path toward aging with grace.

In essence, the vitamins and minerals for anti-aging are more than just capsules and tablets; they are a currency for vitality. Investing in this wealth as part of a holistic lifestyle is perhaps our most prudent venture as we aim to live not just longer lives, but fuller, healthier ones.

Thus, as we continue to unravel the coil of longevity, let us proceed with mindfulness – welcoming a daily dose of these invisible, yet indomitable guardians of our youth. For it is in their subtle, yet pivotal support that we find the nuances of elegance in aging, an experience we're all inherently entitled to.

Herbal Supplements: Benefits and Considerations Navigating the world of herbal supplements can be likened to wandering through an ancient and dense garden – there's a plethora of plants, each with its own tale of healing and health enhancement. For those yearning to age gracefully and uphold vitality, these natural allies often become an integral part of their regimen. However, threading the path efficiently requires a marriage of reverence for tradition and scrutiny through the lens of modern science.

Let's embark on understanding the role of herbal supplements in the anti-aging conquest. Plants such as Ginkgo biloba, Turmeric, and Ashwagandha have been heralded for centuries for their potential to combat the signs of aging. Today, they're not only a testament to anecdotal success but are also increasingly subjected to the empirical gaze, revealing compelling insights into their chemistry and interaction with the human body.

The allure of herbal supplements often lies in their purported ability to address the root causes of aging rather than merely masking symptoms. Take antioxidants, for instance – these natural compounds are central in the fight against free radicals, malicious molecules implicated in cellular aging and dysfunction. Many herbs are rich in these antioxidants, offering a botanical shield against the ravages of time.

But as with all things powerful, herbal supplements come with their caveats. Not all green is gold – potency and purity vary widely, and without careful consideration, one could venture into risky territories. Quality control is still an evolving frontier in the supplement industry, framing the importance of selecting products from reputable sources. Choose poorly, and one may encounter contaminants or ingredients that deviate from the label's promise.

Furthermore, the interaction of these herbal comrades with each other – and with conventional medications – cannot be overlooked. They're part and parcel of a complex biological network within us, and what aids one may ail another. It's critical to consult with healthcare providers, especially when one is on a cocktail of prescription drugs. The interplay between certain herbs and medications could either diminish the efficacy of your treatment or amplify side effects.

Take echinacea, revered for immune support; it might seem like a harmless boost in a capsule. However, for those on immunosuppressive therapy, such as individuals with autoimmune diseases or organ transplants, this immune stimulation could pose a threat. Such nuances underscore the importance of personalized guidance and the principle of 'no one-size-fits-all' in herbal supplementation.

It also begs acknowledgment that, while the benefits of herbal supplements can be striking, patience is an accompanying virtue. Unlike conventional medicine, whose effects can be swift and potent, herbs often espouse a gentler approach. They work subtly, encouraging the body's innate healing mechanisms to tip the scales back to equilibrium. Hence, it's about long-term commitment rather than expecting overnight miracles.

Considering the hormone fluctuations that come with aging, particularly the diminishing tide of estrogen and testosterone, some turn to herbs like Black Cohosh or Maca. Their adaptogenic properties may help smooth the hormonal rollercoaster, but the key lies in their judicious use. Appreciating their gentle nudge rather than a forceful push can make all the difference in how they're integrated into one's lifestyle.

While clinical trials are growing in number, the robust evidence for specific anti-aging benefits of various herbs can still be somewhat spotty. But is the absence of evidence the evidence of absence? Not necessarily. Observational data can't be dismissed, and often, the true gift of herbal supplementation is revealed through consistent, thoughtful usage.

Moreover, for those pondering longevity, it isn't just about adding years to life but adding life to those years. There's an evergreen charm in herbs like Rhodiola that have been mooted to amplify energy levels or St. John's Wort's potential to brighten the dim days of mood swings. Yet, it's paramount to remember that these are mere threads in the tapestry of a holistic lifestyle and not solitary magic bullets.

Age can be more than a mere number; it can bring wisdom, and part of that wisdom is recognizing one's unique physiological narrative. One's genetic makeup, lifestyle, and existing health conditions play starring roles in how well an herbal supplement might integrate and perform within their biological script.

In closing the chapter on herbal supplements, do not let their natural origin lull you into complacency. Due diligence in research, sourcing, and consultation with healthcare professionals is your compass in this lush landscape. The right herbal supplementation could indeed be a pivotal character in your personal anti-aging story, weaving into your daily regimen with potential and poise. As you turn the page, keep in mind that with great power – like that of nature's bounty – comes great responsibility.

Chapter 13:
Alternative Anti-Aging Therapies

A s we edge past the foundational pillars of nutrition, hydration, and exercise that bolster our defenses against time's relentless march, we arrive at a compelling frontier teeming with potential: alternative anti-aging therapies. You're probably seeking out that extra edge, a hidden gem that might unlock more vibrant years. Let's turn over some of these stones together and peer into the world of acupuncture, reflexology, and a plethora of other complementary practices shrouded in both historical mystique and modern curiosity. Imagine a tapestry woven from the threads of ancient tradition and contemporary science—this is precisely the enthralling landscape we're exploring. You deserve to know what might tip the scales in favor of not just prolonged lifespan but amplified vitality. So, let's critically and open-mindedly evaluate the tapestry of treatments that promise rejuvenation beyond the scope of pills and procedures, where the subtleties of energy, balance, and holistic wellness take center stage.

Exploring Acupuncture, Massage, and More As we venture deeper into the realm of anti-aging therapies, there's a treasure trove of wisdom to be unearthed within the practices often labeled as "alternative". Acupuncture and massage therapy, for instance, stand not on the fringes, but rather at the crossroads of ancient traditions and modern science. And they're just a starting point. These forms of therapy open the door to a holistic approach to longevity that complements the body's natural healing capabilities.

Acupuncture, a pillar of traditional Chinese medicine, has intrigued the West with its mysterious yet effective results. It's like a delicate dance of energy, where the practitioner places hair-thin needles at specific points on the body. This is believed to rebalance energy flow—or "qi"—and catalyze the body's healing mechanisms. Studies suggest that acupuncture can help manage chronic pain, a common adversary as we age, and even contribute to improved sleep and reduced stress.

Then, there's the universally beloved massage therapy. It's practically a synonym for relaxation, but its benefits extend far beyond. Kneading muscles and applying pressure doesn't just feel good; it enhances blood circulation, provides pain relief, and can alleviate symptoms of conditions like arthritis—common concerns that escalate with age. Also, let's not overlook the power of touch to soothe the mind and improve mental health—a critical piece of the longevity puzzle.

The spectrum of massage styles is vast, from the gentle strokes of Swedish massage to the targeted pressure of deep tissue work. It's this diversity that equips massage therapy with a broad toolkit to address an equally diverse array of needs that arise as we journey through the years.

Reflexology, another intriguing practice, zeroes in on the feet, hands, and ears, positing that these extremities are a map to the whole body. By manipulating specific areas, reflexologists aim not only to elicit serenity within the soul but also to provoke physiological changes—like better digestion and pain relief—that target aging's common ailments.

Beyond these well-known practices lies a galaxy of other therapies. Think about the soothing warmth of hot stone therapy, the rejuvenating embrace of hydrotherapy, or the gentle stretching of Thai massage. They each offer unique avenues to harness the body's capacity to repair and rejuvenate itself.

Chiropractic care is another modality that, while sometimes controversial, garners a loyal following, thanks to impressions of pain reduction and improved mobility. As vertebrae align and nerves communicate more freely, the body operates more harmoniously—a state that can only benefit our aging vessels.

Aromatherapy makes use of the evocative power of scent to heal. The essential oils used are not just fragrant but functional, each with a specific purpose, from calming anxiety to promoting better sleep—issues that can become more pronounced as the candles on our birthday cakes multiply.

Then there's cupping therapy, with its telltale round bruises that grabbed headlines during the Olympics. It's claimed by enthusiasts to stimulate blood flow and ease muscle tension, though untouched by the same depth of research as acupuncture or massage.

No discussion of alternative therapies is complete without mentioning Reiki, a Japanese technique for stress reduction and relaxation that also promotes healing. It's based on the unseen life force energy that flows through us, and practitioners aim to improve your flow of energy to aid in healing and longevity.

What's truly compelling about these therapies is not just their potential physical benefits, but their tacit acknowledgment that our well-being is about more than the physical. These practices embrace the mental, emotional, and sometimes spiritual aspects of health, vital areas that often escape the microscope of conventional medicine.

One can't expect to plunge into acupuncture or enjoy a weekly massage and suddenly arrest the aging process. These practices are integrative; they're most effective when part of a multifaceted approach to wellness that includes a balanced diet, regular exercise, and good sleep hygiene. They're about enhancing quality of life, about making the golden years gleam that bit brighter.

Before we uncork the little-known wonders of evidence-based complementary practices in the next section, it's essential to understand that the efficacy of therapies like acupuncture, massage, and their kin vary from person to person. What might act as a panacea for one may be mere placebo for another.

It's also about personal preference. Some might find the idea of needles unsettling and thus, won't relax enough to allow acupuncture to work, whereas others could view it as the highlight of their week. It's this subjectivity that underscores the importance of trying different therapies and observing what resonates with your own body and mind.

In the ballet of aging, your own preferences, experiences, and beliefs will shape the choreography of your self-care routine—whether it includes the firm pressure of a massage or the delicate touch of an acupuncturist's needle. The key is to listen to and honor what your body tells you, because in the symphony of life, every individual requires a unique harmony of care.

So, in contemplating this tapestry of therapies, each woven with tradition and gilded with possibilities, it's worth experimenting, with an open mind and a listening body. In the next chapter, we'll unravel the threads of evidence-based complementary practices, offering a glimpse into what science says about these storied modalities and how they align with our quest for longevity.

Evidence-Based Complementary Practices weave into the tapestry of anti-aging strategies like threads of gold, elevating the overall picture of well-being. While we've covered the spectrum from nutrition to hydration, and stress management to sleep, there's a dimension that health enthusiasts often, quite mistakenly, gloss over: the realm of complementary practices. These practices not only add richness to our anti-aging regimen but deserve serious consideration for their evidence-backed benefits.

Let's begin with a cornerstone of complementary health care—meditation. You may have heard of its calming effects, but did you know that meditation can physiologically reverse stress-related changes in genes linked to poor health and depression? That's right, consistent meditative practices can literally change your gene expression, veering you on a cellular level towards longevity and health. Over time, meditation enhances brain gray matter, improving memory, attention, and resilience to stress. It's a practice grounded in millennia of tradition, yet it's backed by today's cutting-edge science.

Moving onto the physical plane, yoga, often viewed as the perfect harmony of body and mind, merits a closer look for its anti-aging prowess. It goes beyond flexibility and balance, with studies exhibiting its potency in reducing systemic inflammation, a notorious accomplice in the aging process. As an added boon, some forms of yoga induce a relaxation response that can lower blood pressure and enhance cardiac health—a major win in the quest for longevity.

Speaking of relaxation, let's talk about tai chi, a martial art turned meditative practice. It's like a slow dance with your health, where the measured movements help maintain joint flexibility, boost cognitive function, and manage stress. In the elderly, tai chi has been shown to reduce the risk of falls, a critical factor in maintaining independence and preventing age-related injuries. Its low-impact nature renders it a sustainable exercise for all ages and fitness levels, embodying the gentle approach one might take towards lifelong health maintenance.

The use of herbs and botanicals also shines in the compendium of anti-aging strategies. Take, for example, turmeric—the golden spice that's not just for flavoring your curry. Curcumin, the active component in turmeric, harbors potent anti-inflammatory and antioxidant properties. It's been linked to enhanced cognitive function and a reduced risk of several age-related diseases. However, to truly reap curcumin's benefits, one might need to pair it with black pepper to enhance its bioavailability.

Acupuncture, with its roots in traditional Chinese medicine, punctuates the importance of body energy flow or 'qi' for health and longevity. Now, even western science acknowledges acupuncture's efficacy for pain relief, one of the common maladies that can plague our later years. It's believed that acupuncture can stimulate the nervous system and release certain neurotransmitters that modulate pain and promote a sense of well-being.

Another practice gaining ground is massage therapy—a method not just for relaxation but for its therapeutic effects on the body. Regular massage has been associated with reduced stiffness and pain, improved circulation, and even enhanced immune function. Particularly, for those advancing in years, massage may be an excellent tool for managing chronic pain and improving quality of life.

Aromatic essential oils, used wisely, can create ambiances conducive to stress relief and relaxation. Lavender oil, for instance, has been linked to improved sleep quality—an essential part of any anti-aging routine. Meanwhile, peppermint oil might invigorate the senses and improve concentration. The key to using essential oils is understanding their properties and integrating them thoughtfully into your daily practices.

Let's not forget the healing power of music. Sure, it's great for entertainment, but music therapy has emerged as a bona fide adjunct to improving various health outcomes. From reducing stress and improving mood to enhancing cognitive function in people with dementia, music can be a delightful and non-invasive add-on to our longevity toolkit.

Chiropractic care has also carved out a legitimate place in the field of anti-aging. By adjusting misalignments in the spine, chiropractors can reduce pain, improve mobility, and even impact nervous system function. And let's face it, maintaining a healthy, pain-free back is crucial for an active, joyful life at any age.

Art and expression come next, often underrated in their impact on health. Engaging in creative activities has been linked to improved mental health, reduced stress, and a sharper brain. Whether it's painting, writing, or sculpting, creative expression is not just a hobby—it's a way to keep the brain plastic and youthful.

Grounding or earthing, which involves direct skin contact with the ground, is an emerging trend based on the idea that connecting with the Earth's natural charge can impact health. Preliminary research suggests that it might reduce inflammation and oxidative stress. Walking barefoot on grass or sand might just reconnect you to nature's healing potential.

Let's circle back to the dietary realm to address fermented foods such as yogurt, kombucha, and kefir. These aren't your average snacks; they're probiotic powerhouses that support gut health—a crucial factor in overall well-being and immunity. The gut microbiome is intimately linked to various aspects of health, including inflammation, which as we've learned, plays a significant role in aging.

Biofeedback is another technique that epitomizes the union of technology and wellness. By using electronic monitoring to convey information about physiological processes, individuals can learn to control bodily functions that were thought to be involuntarily, like heart rate or muscle tension. This control has profound implications for managing stress and its age-accelerating effects.

Last but not least, we must mention hydration, touched upon in an earlier chapter, as one of the most foundational yet overlooked elements of anti-aging. Water is not just about quenching thirst—it's about supporting every cellular process in our body. From aiding digestion to maintaining skin elasticity, proper hydration is perhaps the most accessible and impactful practice we can adopt for longevity.

In conclusion, your anti-aging regime doesn't have to be a monotonous script of diet and exercise. Sprinkle in these evidence-based complementary practices to enrich your quest for longevity and vitality. They are not merely alternative options to conventional wisdom; they are integral components of a sophisticated, well-rounded approach to aging gracefully and healthily. Just as a seasoned chef uses a variety of spices to create a culinary masterpiece, so too can you mix these practices into your life for a rich, vibrant, and prolonged existence.

Chapter 14:
Detoxification for Longevity

As we continue to delve into the myriad aspects of slowing down the hands of time, we encounter the principle of detoxification—a powerhouse in our quest for longevity. Imagine our bodies as complex networks of highways, bustling with the traffic of nutrients and waste. Just as roadways can become congested, our bodies, too, can be burdened by toxins that impede optimal function. But here's the kicker: detoxing isn't about drastic cleanses that leave you famished. It's about enhancing your body's natural cleaning systems to operate more efficiently. We're talking about a sensible, science-supported approach to ridding your life of dietary and environmental pollutants, which, if left unchecked, can contribute to the acceleration of the aging process. So let's clear the air—and our bodies—with strategies that reinforce our biological resilience, ensuring that our internal engines run cleaner and longer, well into the golden years.

Cleansing Your Body for Better Health As we traverse the journey of aging gracefully, we scrutinize various components that contribute to a robust and vibrant life. A particularly intriguing chapter in this odyssey is the concept of cleansing our body. The notion that we can, in a sense, "reset" our internal environment is alluring and, in many ways, reflects our desire for renewal.

Starting off, it's essential to understand why our bodies might need cleansing. Day in and day out, the human body is subjected to an array of toxins from our diet, environment, and even the air we breathe. These toxins can accumulate over time, potentially hampering our metabolic pathways and putting additional stress on organs like the liver and kidneys.

The goal of a body cleanse, then, is to assist these organs in their natural detoxification processes. It's about creating an optimal environment for them to do their job more effectively. You could think of it as taking a load off or giving these systems a "vacation" so they can return to work rejuvenated.

Let's touch upon our daily diet, which plays a critical role in this process. A diet rich in fruits, vegetables, whole grains, and lean proteins provides a plethora of nutrients that aid in the detoxification process. Antioxidants found in these foods are powerhouses when it comes to neutralizing harmful free radicals caused by toxin exposure.

Hydration cannot be overstated either. Water plays a pivotal role in nearly every bodily function, and when it comes to cleansing, it helps flush out unwanted substances. We talked about optimizing hydration earlier, and when paired with a balanced diet, the stage is perfectly set for your natural detox systems to operate at their peak.

Another significant method involves liver support. Your liver is the ultimate multitasker, filtering out toxins and breaking them down. Foods that are known to promote liver health include those high in compounds such as sulfur —think garlic and onions — and those with liver-friendly vitamins and minerals, like leafy green vegetables.

Physical activity, which is discussed in depth in another chapter, also plays a supporting role in cleansing our bodies. Regular exercise increases blood flow, which helps carry away waste products. Moreover, sweating, which occurs during exercise, is another way your body can eliminate toxins.

The often-overlooked aspect of cleansing is sleep. Quality sleep allows our brain to carry out a unique type of cleansing process, removing toxic byproducts that accumulate throughout the day. This "brainwashing" is crucial as it is implicated in maintaining cognitive function, as we'll explore in the chapters concerning brain health.

We must acknowledge that our bodies are designed to cleanse themselves and that a balanced lifestyle supports this natural mechanism. Extreme detoxes and cleanses often marketed to us may sound tempting, but caution and skepticism are in order. The question begs to be asked: Are these intense detox protocols as beneficial as the rhythms of a steady, balanced lifestyle?

The truth lies in moderation and evidence-based practices. Incorporating periods of fasting, for example, has been shown to have benefits in cellular repair processes, but such practices should be approached responsibly and ideally under the guidance of a healthcare professional. We delve into safe and effective detox methods later on, steering clear of fads and focusing on sustainable health.

Stress, an ever-present force in modern life, is another aspect we can't ignore. Its involvement in the aging process is covered in depth in our discussions on stress management. Stress can disrupt our body's natural detox processes, so managing it becomes integral to maintaining balance. Through tactics like mindful meditation and yoga, we can support our body's ability to cleanse itself by reducing the toll stress takes on us.

Supplementation, discussed in an earlier chapter, also ties into the cleansing conversation. Cleanse-friendly supplements like milk thistle, known for its liver-protective qualities, and high-fiber powders can complement a cleansing diet. Nevertheless, indiscriminate use of supplements without professional advice could lead to more harm than benefit.

Moving beyond the transactional nature of "cleansing" products, we arrive at a holistic approach to bodily purification. It encompasses everything from the air we breathe to the thoughts we entertain. Ensuring a toxin-reducing environment can be as important as the foods and liquids we ingest. Practices like using air purifiers and choosing natural cleaning products reduce our toxic load with each breath and each touch.

As we come to terms with the complexity of our body's systems, it becomes evident that cleanses are not quick fixes. They are part of a larger picture of health. Longevity isn't just about adding years to life, but adding life to those years, and this includes thinking about our body's needs holistically and sustainably.

Ultimately, cleansing your body for better health isn't about drastic measures or harsh regimens. It's about respecting the intricate machinery of your body and aiding it in functioning at its full potential. With a mix of mindful diet, exercise, stress management, and overall lifestyle choices, we pave the way for a cleaner, more vibrant self. And this path leads us not just toward longevity but toward a life rich in vitality and exuberance.

Safe and Effective Detox Methods Moving through life, the idea of detoxification often bubbles up with the promise of renewed vitality and health—a tempting prospect as we journey through the aging process. It brings forth an image of flushing out the old to make way for the new and rejuvenated. But let's navigate through this with eyes wide open and understand that the landscape of detox methods is as varied as it is controversial.

Firstly, let's recognize that our bodies are elegantly designed to detoxify naturally. The liver, kidneys, lungs, and even our skin are in constant modes of cleansing. However, our modern environment sometimes floods us with more toxins than our bodies can handle efficiently. So how do we aid our bodies without falling into potentially harmful fads? Well, moderation and evidence-based practices are key.

One of the most accessible and scientifically supported ways to enhance your body's detoxification process is through hydration. Upping your intake of clear, clean water helps to flush toxins through your kidneys, and aids in every cellular function. It's not about chugging gallons but being consistent with sipping water throughout the day.

Switching to a diet high in fiber is also a brilliant move. Fiber-rich foods like vegetables, fruits, and whole grains speed up the elimination process in your digestive tract, and make sure toxins aren't sticking around longer than they're welcome. They bind to the bad stuff and help sweep it out the door—figuratively speaking, of course.

Another detox method that's making waves for the right reasons is regular exercise. When you get moving, you increase blood circulation, and that helps ferry toxins to the proper channels for elimination. Plus, don't discount the power of sweating it out. You're not just burning calories; you're also releasing toxins through your pores.

Speaking of elimination pathways, saunas have a tradition for detox that's backed by modern science. Sauna bathing aids in toxin elimination through deep sweat. Just make sure you're adequately hydrated and listen to your body to avoid overheating.

While it may not be the first thing that comes to mind, quality sleep is a detox hero. During sleep, your brain essentially 'takes out the trash' through a process known as the glymphatic system. It's like the nocturnal clean-up crew for your central nervous system, so ensuring you get enough rest aids this vital process.

From an herbal standpoint, milk thistle stands tall. It's not a fix-all, but it can assist liver function, which is your main detox engine. Before delving into the world of herbal supplements, though, always consult with a healthcare provider to ensure they're appropriate for your personal health context.

Then, there's the trend of juice cleanses which can sometimes do more harm than good by depriving your body of necessary nutrients and disrupting your metabolic balance. Instead of going to extremes, incorporating detoxifying green juices as part of a balanced diet could offer some benefits without the associated risks.

A detox method that's often overlooked is mindful stress management. Chronic stress can wreak havoc on your body's natural detox abilities by weakening your immune system and slowing down the detoxification enzymes in your liver. Techniques like deep-breathing exercises, yoga, or meditation can be powerful allies in maintaining an effective internal cleansing system.

Don't forget about your skin! Dry brushing has been touted for its ability to stimulate the lymphatic system, which plays a crucial role in detoxification. Gentle, circular brush movements not only exfoliate but also help in moving toxins through your lymphatic pathways for processing and elimination.

On the subject of skin, alternating hot and cold showers is another method believed to stimulate circulation and aid detoxification. By contracting and dilating blood vessels, this practice might help move toxins more efficiently through the blood. It's invigorating, to say the least, but remember to exercise caution if you have cardiovascular concerns.

Probiotics and prebiotics also deserve mention. These gut-friendly additives support a healthy microbiome, which is pivotal for proper digestion and toxin removal. Foods rich in these elements, or high-quality supplements, can make a difference in your body's detoxifying prowess. However, as with any supplement, it's wise to chat with your doctor before starting a new regimen.

Teas, particularly green and dandelion, are often recommended for their potential detoxifying effects. They're rich in antioxidants and have diuretic properties, which help in flushing out waste. But moderation is key—excessive consumption can lead to other health issues.

In contrast to these gentle, supportive methods, we should tread carefully around 'detox' products that promise instant results. Quick fixes are not only often ineffective but might also introduce other stressors to your system. It's crucial to approach detox with a long-game mindset; it's less about dramatic purges and more about consistent, healthy practices that support your body's intrinsic pathways.

Finally, it's worth noting that your environment—both personal and global—affects your body's toxin load. Using non-toxic, eco-friendly products in your home can reduce overall exposure, lessening the burden on your detox pathways. Small shifts can result in significant long-term health benefits.

In conclusion, safe and effective detox methods are those that enhance your body's natural processes, provide steady support, and integrate seamlessly into a healthy lifestyle. There's no magic bullet for detox, but with these sensible strategies, we can assist our bodies in doing what they do best—protecting, healing, and rejuvenating themselves.

Chapter 15:
Advances in Anti-Aging Medicine

As we've seen, the journey towards longevity is paved with deliberate choices, from nutrient-rich diets to restorative sleep. Treading further into the realm of possibilities, we arrive at a fascinating juncture—advances in anti-aging medicine are reshaping our expectations of the golden years. It's here that the borders between the once-distant future and our present reality become intriguingly blurred. Cutting-edge treatments, once the fodder of science fiction, are emerging with the promise to not only decelerate aging but to repair and rejuvenate on a cellular level. This chapter dives into groundbreaking therapies like senolytics that selectively target senescent cells, peptide bioregulators that can reboot cellular function, and the potential of gene editing tools like CRISPR to prevent age-related diseases. Yet, with great power comes great responsibility, and with each scientific leap, ethical conundrums follow closely. We'll weigh the breakthroughs against their societal impacts, fostering a discussion that remains anchored in a humanistic approach to health and longevity. It's not about chasing immortality; it's about enriching the quality of every moment we have.

Exploring Cutting-Edge Treatments As we turn the page from understanding the basic principles that safeguard our youthfulness, we now dive into the riveting realm of avant-garde treatments that are redefining the limits of our life's timeline. The domain of cutting-edge treatments is teeming with innovation, where scientists and researchers are the new pioneers on the frontier of age defiance.

Imagine a world where we could simply erase the biological markers of aging, like smoothing wrinkles out of a linen shirt. In that world, lab coats and bio-tech labs replace fountains and their mythical promises of youth. It's a reality coming into focus thanks to the relentless pursuit of medical advancement. Here, we're not just talking about surface-level solutions; we're talking about fundamentally altering how our bodies age at the cellular and molecular level.

To set the stage, let's first recognize a groundbreaking shift in aging interventions: the use of stem cells. Once the stuff of science fiction, stem cell therapies are now bringing forth regenerative possibilities that many thought impossible. The ability to replace or rejuvenate damaged tissues offers not just enhanced longevity but also the quality of life we all yearn for as we age.

Adjacent to stem cell therapies is the exciting field of gene editing, specifically CRISPR-Cas9 technology. It's as if we've been granted a molecular pair of scissors, allowing us to snip away genetic predispositions to certain age-related diseases. The potential here is monumental, raising both hope and ethical questions. We can't bypass a discussion on tweaking the blueprints of life without addressing the responsibilities that come with such power.

Peptide therapies are another contender in the anti-aging arena. These short chains of amino acids are showing promise in enhancing tissue repair and modulating immune responses. Administered correctly, peptides could help our bodies resist the wear and tear of time.

Then, there's the burgeoning area of senolytics—drugs specifically designed to target and eliminate senescent cells, those that have stopped dividing and contribute to aging and age-related diseases. By clearing out these cellular "zombies," we may be able to reduce inflammation and restore vitality to aging tissues. It's a pharmaceutical take on the age-old fantasy of the cleansing elixir.

An interesting dimension to the tapestry of modern treatments is the concept of bioprinting—the layer-by-layer creation of tissue that could one day lead to the printing of whole organs. Bioprinting harnesses the precision of 3D printing to address one of aging's critical problems—the failure of organs. This isn't just a lifeline for those awaiting transplants; it's a potential game-changer in extending human healthspan.

Among the potential elixirs of youth are the sirtuin-activating compounds (STACs). These molecules can imitate caloric restriction, a known method for extending lifespan in various organisms. By activating the sirtuin pathways associated with aging, these compounds could unlock natural mechanisms in our own cells that promote longevity.

As we peer deeper into our own biology, the microbiome surfaces as a critical player in aging. The trillions of microorganisms residing in and on us influence our health profoundly. By understanding and manipulating these communities, particularly through microbiome transplants, we can potentially stave off diseases that come with aging and optimize our body's functionality.

Wouldn't it be something if we could charge our cells like we do our phones? That's the promise of mitochondrial optimization therapies. Our cellular powerhouses, the mitochondria, decline in function as we age. By targeting them with specific treatments, we might be able to reinvigorate our cells, keeping them energetic and, by extension, keeping us more vibrant.

Another foray into future treatment is the use of nanotechnology—tiny robots and particles designed to repair or even replace cellular components, or to deliver drugs precisely where they're needed. This microscopic army could become a mainstay in the battle against the deterioration of aging.

Meanwhile, neuroplasticity enhancement suggests that we can teach an old brain new tricks. Through cognitive training and perhaps soon with pharmacological assistance, there's potential to strengthen the brain's resilience against degeneration, keeping our minds as nimble as our rejuvenated bodies.

With longevity comes the increased risk of cancer, but onco-geriatrics intersects anti-aging and cancer treatments. New therapies that target cancer cells without harming healthy ones preserve the body's integrity for a longer period of time—offering a beacon of hope in what was once a grim diagnosis for an aging population.

Artificial intelligence isn't just for self-driving cars; it's entering the medical field with gusto. AI-driven diagnostics, treatment plans, and even predictive modeling for age-related diseases may soon be the norm. Such precision medicine will allow treatments to be tailored to individual profiles, revolutionizing our approach to health care as we age.

Lest we assume all innovations are high-tech, let's consider the role of nutraceuticals—a blend of nutrition and pharmaceutical. Certain compounds found in foods, when concentrated and administered as supplements, might offer protective benefits against the ravages of time. Imagine harnessing the power of natural compounds to not just nourish, but to heal and preserve our bodies.

In conclusion, the future is already at our doorstep, with therapies once considered the wild musings of optimistic futurists now entering clinical trials and some even making their way into medical practice. The quest for longevity isn't a horizon we pursue aimlessly—it's a tangible destination, adorned with the beacons of scientific discovery. This exploration into cutting-edge treatments is not just a patchwork of hope; it's a testament to human ingenuity and the relentless pursuit of not just more years in our life, but more life in our years.

Ethics and the Future of Anti-Aging Therapies Undeniably, the quest to halt or even reverse the aging process is as ancient as human civilization itself. The fountain of youth, said to restore the vitality of anyone who drinks or bathes in its waters, is a myth that underscores humanity's deep-seated desire for perpetual youth. However, as modern science edges closer to making substantial breakthroughs in anti-aging therapies, we're compelled to navigate the treacherous waters of ethical considerations.

In the sphere of anti-aging, treatments are emerging that challenge our traditional understanding of aging as an inevitable process. From regenerative medicine to genetic tinkering, science is opening doors to possibilities that were once confined to the realm of science fiction. But with these advancements, we must ask ourselves critical ethical questions. Who gets access to these therapies? At what cost? And what are the implications for society at large?

The potential for exacerbating social inequalities is one ethical quandary we can't ignore. Imagine a world where only the affluent can afford treatments to look and feel younger for decades longer than their less wealthy counterparts. The gap between the haves and have-nots could widen dramatically, not just in terms of financial resources, but also in health and lifespan.

Then there is the consideration of fairness in the allocation of limited resources. If anti-aging treatments prove to require significant medical resources or a financial investment that could be spent on other public health initiatives, we must scrutinize whether these treatments should become a priority. Is it more ethical to direct these resources toward treatments that extend the healthy period of midlife, or should we focus on curing diseases that afflict the young and rob them of the chance to live a full life?

We must also consider the environmental impact of a population that lives significantly longer. Earth's resources are already under strain, and a surge in population longevity could amplify existing issues like overpopulation, resource scarcity, and environmental degradation. The ethical stewardship of our planet necessitates a discourse on how anti-aging therapies fit into the larger picture of sustainability.

Social and familial structures could also feel the weight of longevity. When multiple generations live longer, potentially healthier lives, it redefines concepts like retirement and eldercare. How will increasing lifespans affect the job market, career development, and the dynamics within households and communities?

Personal identity and psychological well-being are also at play when longevity extends. Our sense of self is partially determined by life's stages. If those stages are drastically altered or extended, individuals might grapple with new challenges related to their identity and purpose, potentially leading to unforeseen psychological implications.

The medical profession's oath to 'do no harm' takes on new layers of complexity when discussing anti-aging. As treatments advance, medical professionals must distinguish between interventions that promise true health benefits and those that risk the wellness of individuals for the sake of cosmetic enhancements or dubious life-extending promises.

Furthermore, extended lifespans could have profound implications on population-wide health dynamics. If anti-aging therapies decrease the incidence of age-related diseases, this would shift healthcare needs significantly. Conversely, if they merely extend life without improving health, we could see an increase in older individuals requiring long-term medical care, adding stress to healthcare systems.

Hence, what anti-aging therapy developers and proponents advocate for goes beyond science; it borders on societal philosophy. The vision of living longer must be accompanied by the vision of living well, and doing so in a manner that embraces the collective well-being of all citizens.

Amidst all this, the role of regulation and oversight cannot be understated. Robust ethical guidelines and regulations must be developed and enforced to ensure that anti-aging therapies are safe, effective, and within the bounds of moral social conduct. The seductive allure of immortality should not blind us to the need for rigorous scientific validation and ethical responsibility.

In the same breath, we must also think about consent and autonomy. As much as society needs to grapple with the wider implications of anti-aging, on a personal level, individuals must have the autonomy to make informed decisions about their health and body, free from coercion or unrealistic expectations set by societal standards of beauty and success.

Collaboration across disciplines – joining ethicists, scientists, policymakers, and the public – will be critical to addressing these concerns. A well-rounded, deeply contemplated approach to anti-aging will likely yield the most equitable and positive outcomes for our society. It's about nurturing a culture of wisdom that respects the natural processes, but also embraces responsible innovation.

In crafting the future of anti-aging therapies, we are also shaping the trajectory of human civilization. The implications ripple across every aspect of life, from individual choices to global policies. As much as we chart these unexplored waters, we must do so with a profound sense of responsibility, ensuring that the tide of progress lifts all ships, not just the yachts.

Ultimately, as we gaze into the horizon of our potentially extended futures, we see more than the promise of longevity. We see the reflection of our values, the illumination of our integrity, and the silhouette of the society we aspire to be. Anti-aging is not just a topic confined to clinic doors or research labs; it's a catalyst for a broad-ranging social and moral discourse. In this sense, the future of anti-aging therapies is as much about ethics as it is about scientific breakthroughs – a delicate balance that we must strive to maintain as we look toward a longer, healthier, and more equitable future for all.

Chapter 16:
Personalized Medicine and Aging

Diving into the world of personalized medicine, we find ourselves at the fascinating intersection where cutting-edge technology meets the timeless quest for longevity. Imagine a future where your medical care is tailored specifically to your genetic makeup, lifestyle, and even your environment. That future is now. In this chapter, we'll unpack how personalized medicine is transforming the way we approach aging. From designer supplements to customized diet plans, we'll explore how uncovering your unique DNA blueprint can unlock the secrets to a longer and healthier life. You'll learn about the role of genetic testing and how it paves the way for targeted interventions that can slow down the clock on aging, reducing the risk of age-related diseases, and redefining what it means to grow older with vitality. Sure, you can't change your genes, but with the right knowledge, you can learn to play them like a symphony, hitting the right notes for optimal health as you age.

Tailoring Health Strategies to Your DNA Imagine harnessing the intricate blueprint of your DNA, a vast and personal database, to craft the ultimate health strategy tailored just for you. For centuries, healthcare has been a one-size-fits-all affair. But as science zooms in on the relation between genes and longevity, it opens up a thrilling possibility: What if you could optimize your lifestyle to complement your genetic predispositions and edge closer to that fabled fountain of youth?

Let's dive a bit deeper into the genetic pool. Your DNA contains genes—sections of code—that influence how quickly (or slowly) you age, how your body responds to different foods, how robust your immune system might be, and your vulnerability to specific diseases. When we talk about personalizing health strategies, it's about making your genetic tendencies your allies instead of your foes.

This is not sci-fi—it's science. Genetic testing has leaped out of the realms of academia and into the public sphere. Now, with a simple saliva sample, you can unlock the secrets buried in your DNA. The results? They can speak volumes about your optimal diet, how your body processes vitamins and minerals, and even your ideal type of exercise. Yet, having the information is only the starting line; understanding and implementing it is the real race.

Take nutrition, for instance. Say your genetic test reveals a higher risk for celiac disease, a disorder causing adverse reactions to gluten. Armed with this knowledge, you could preemptively adapt a gluten-free diet. Or maybe, your genes suggest you're less likely to metabolize vitamin D efficiently. In this case, soaking in a bit more sunshine and supplementing with vitamin D could be your key to maintaining bone health and warding off potential deficiencies.

When it comes to exercise, our genetic makeup influences not just our potential for muscle development but also how our bodies respond to different types of physical activity. Some of us are naturally endowed marathon runners, while others are sprinters. Knowing your genetic predisposition can help tailor your workout routine to maximize health benefits while minimizing injury risks.

But here's the thing: genetics is a piece of the puzzle, not the entire picture. Your lifestyle, environment, and personal decisions weave together with your DNA to create your health narrative. While you can't change your genetic code, you can change many of these other factors. Understanding your genetics empowers you to make more informed choices, but it does not predetermine your destiny.

Now, addressing the elephant in the room: privacy and ethics. With the rise of genetic testing, concerns about privacy and data security are legitimate. Your genetic information is personal and sensitive, and how it's used extends beyond your individual health strategies. It's important to work with reputable companies that prioritize your privacy and safeguard your data.

All this gene talk may also ring the bells of inequality. Not everyone has the same access to genetic testing and personalized medicine—yet. Bridging this gap is important so that we can all benefit from these advances, not just a privileged few. Social responsibility must walk hand in hand with scientific progress.

It's also crucial to have a professional interpret your genetic results. While we're making strides in the field, it's still in its adolescence. We're unlocking secrets, but there are plenty more mysteries hidden within our helixes. A genetic counselor can guide you through the data labyrinth, helping you make sense of your results and how they might translate into actionable health decisions.

Moving from the lab to your living room, how does this all fold into daily life? Let's say you've gotten your report back, and it indicates a predisposition for slow metabolism. You might opt for more frequent, smaller meals throughout your day, coupled with high-intensity interval training (HIIT), to rev up that metabolic engine. If your genes suggest a penchant for stress resilience, that doesn't give you the green card to embrace a high-stress lifestyle. Instead, you could use that trait to your advantage, by embarking on careers or roles that others might find too stressful but which you can navigate with more ease.

There's an art to combining the story told by your genes with the one you compose through your choices. It's a dance of nature and nurture. Your DNA lays out a sprawling map of potential roads you can take, but it's the daily steps—the foods you eat, the stress you manage, the sleep you prioritize—that determine the path you walk.

So, before we close this genetic chapter and venture onward, let's commit to the idea that while our genetic heritage is a compass, it's not our fate sealed in stone. We can chart a course toward longevity that respects our innate predispositions without being ruled by them. Genes might load the gun, but lifestyle pulls the trigger—a principle that is empowering, humbling, and invigorating all at once.

Now, while tailoring health strategies to your DNA may sound like the ultimate customization, it's important to remember that it's still a burgeoning field. There are nuances, and there will be trial and error. Customization does not equal perfection, but it does mean progression. Integrating this personalized approach into our lives is a complex but profoundly human endeavor, connecting us with the very essence of our being—our DNA.

With the close of this section on DNA-specific health strategies, we're not just turning a page in a book; we're turning a corner in our health journeys. Embrace the insights that genetics offer, let them inform your choices, and always balance them with the rich tapestry of lifestyle factors that influence aging. Now, let's step into the realm of genetic testing and see how these scientific breakthroughs are becoming accessible tools for shaping our longevity.

The Rise of Genetic Testing As we delve further into personalized medicine, a key innovator emerges that is reshaping our approach to health and aging: genetic testing. It's not just about solving the riddle of our ancestry anymore. Today, genetic consumerism is getting intimate with our DNA, serving up insights that can herald revolutionary strides in precision wellness and the anti-aging crusade.

Imagine a world where instead of one-size-fits-all health recommendations, you're handed a blueprint of your body's strengths, weaknesses, and propensities. That is the lofty promise of genetic testing in the context of aging. Armed with knowledge about how our genes can affect the aging process, we can make informed decisions and tailor strategies that potentially slow down our biological clocks.

But where did this momentum come from? To appreciate the rise in genetic testing, it's key to understand the milestones that have brought us to this point. The completion of the Human Genome Project early in the 21st century was nothing short of a watershed moment—decoding the entire human genetic makeup was like getting the secret recipe to humanity's inner workings.

Now that genetic testing has become more accessible and affordable, droves of individuals are lining up to glean information from their genetic code. Companies are offering kits that provide insights into genetic predispositions for a multitude of conditions and traits, many of which play key roles in the aging process.

We can't talk about aging without touching on chronic diseases. It's common knowledge that the risk of developing conditions like heart disease, diabetes, or Alzheimer's increases with age. Genetic testing can unveil risk factors etched in our DNA, giving us the chance to mitigate these risks with tailored dietary, lifestyle, and medical interventions.

The science behind genetic testing isn't just about preventative measures though; it's also about optimizing well-being. Nutrigenomics, for example, is a burgeoning field that explores how our genes interact with our diet. It's no stretch to say that in the near future, personalized nutrition plans aligned with our genetic profiles could become standard practice for anti-aging lifestyle design.

Connect the dots between genetic markers and exercise, and you get a frontier known as exercise genomics. It suggests the tantalizing possibility that different individuals might be better suited to specific types of workouts, not just based on personal preference, but on their genetic makeup. Targeted exercise regimens, shaped by our genetic dispositions, could thus enhance our vitality and longevity more effectively than general advice.

It's important we address the elephant in the room—privacy concerns and ethical dilemmas are part and parcel with the surge in genetic testing. As beneficial as this technology is, it does open a Pandora's box. Who owns this genetic data? How is it safeguarded? Could it be used against us, say, by insurance companies or employers? These questions bubble to the surface, reminding us that with great power comes great responsibility.

Moreover, there's an undercurrent of skepticism about the applicability of genetic test results. Detractors argue that genetics is only part of the longevity puzzle. Indeed, our environment, habits, and sheer serendipity collaborate with our genes in a complex dance that writes the story of our aging process. The influence of genetics, while undeniable, isn't absolute. This underscores the need for balanced perspectives when incorporating genetic data into anti-aging plans.

Despite potential pitfalls, the allure of personalized medicine through genetic testing is undeniable for the health-conscious individual. It presents an unprecedented opportunity to move beyond guesswork. To take the reins of our health journey with a confidence that is grounded not in hopeful estimations, but in the bedrock of our own biological narrative.

Scientists are laboring tirelessly to untangle the intricate genetic threads that influence our longevity. Such research holds promise for future interventions that could someday extend healthy lifespans. Discoveries like longevity genes in certain populations point to genetic factors that contribute markedly to a longer and healthier life.

Even as we marvel at the potential of genetic testing, it's prudent to maintain a level head. This technology, as dazzling as it is, serves as a tool—not a crystal ball. It empowers us to make sharper decisions and adopt a proactive stance on health but requires judicious interpretation by professionals who can help navigate the nuances of our genetic readouts.

Furthermore, we can leverage the insights gleaned from our genes to personalize other aspects of the anti-aging battleplan—not just in terms of what we eat and how we move our bodies, but how we manage stress, detoxify, and even socialize. Each gene carries a thread in the tapestry of our well-being, awaiting to be woven into a personalized lifestyle that is both scientific and holistic in nature.

Embracing the potential of genetic testing also means engaging with the ethical considerations and controversies that surround its use. A dialogue that includes not only scientists and medical professionals but also ethicists, legislators, and the public must continue to evolve. It's crucial that as we harness the science of our genes to pursue an ageless existence, we do so with an eye on the broader implications for society and individual rights.

In conclusion, the rise of genetic testing in the realm of anti-aging is a testament to humanity's relentless pursuit of knowledge and mastery over its own destiny. As we venture further into uncharted territory, our approach must be grounded in wisdom and foresight. After all, the quest for longevity is not just about adding years to life but about infusing those years with quality and purpose—guided by the very blueprints that make us who we are.

Chapter 17:
Mindfulness and Meditation

As we weave through the tapestry of our lives, marked by the chapters before, we come upon a gentle yet transformative practice: mindfulness and meditation. These time-honored strategies for calming the storm within don't just ease our daily stresses; they're like a tonic for the soul, potentially rewinding the aging clock. The art of being fully present, accompanied by the deep, rhythmic breathing of meditation, has been shown to create a fortress of calm in your mind, meriting a place in your anti-aging arsenal. By deploying these techniques, you're not just indulging in moments of serenity; you're initiating a positive cascade that benefits your entire biological being. Moreover, these practices may bolster our cognitive reserves, building a mental resilience that can weather the tempest of time. It's more than clearing your mind—it's about enriching your life's journey with peace and clarity. In this chapter, you'll discover how to seamlessly fuse mindfulness and meditation into the very fabric of your daily life, ensuring that each breath you take is a step towards a more vibrant and sustainable future.

Techniques for Inner Peace and Longevity Once we have ventured through the avenues of physical well-being—from the impact of hydration to the importance of sleep—it's time to turn inward. Beyond our bodies, the tranquility of our minds profoundly influences longevity. The adage 'mind over matter' isn't just a catchy phrase; it embodies a truth about the human condition that resonates through the ages.

In this conversation about inner peace, it's essential to acknowledge that stress isn't just an uncomfortable emotion—it's a physical state that can wreak havoc on our bodies. Chronic stress accelerates aging at the cellular level, so managing it isn't a luxury—it's a necessity. The techniques we'll explore aren't just fluff; they're backed by robust research that points to their efficacy in elongating life by not just years, but healthy, vibrant years.

Let's start with meditation. Often misunderstood as a mystical practice reserved for monks and hermits, meditation is actually a scientifically supported method for reducing stress and improving health. At its core, meditation is about focusing the mind and finding a sense of stillness amid the chaos of life. This isn't about turning off your thoughts—it's about observing them without judgment. Consistent meditation can lower blood pressure, decrease anxiety, and even slow the aging process by reducing the shortening of telomeres, the protective caps on the ends of chromosomes.

Breathing exercises, though seemingly simple, are another powerful tool at our disposal. When we're stressed, our breath becomes shallow and rapid. By consciously slowing and deepening our breath, we can activate the body's relaxation response. One method, known as the 4-7-8 technique, involves inhaling for four counts, holding the breath for seven counts, and exhaling for eight. This rhythmic breathing can help steady the heartbeat and signal to the brain that it's time to unwind.

Yoga, a practice that marries breath and movement, serves as more than just a form of exercise; it's a conduit to longevity. The physical postures, or asanas, keep the body flexible and strong, while the meditative aspects promote mental clarity and stress relief. Studies have shown that those who practice yoga regularly can experience reductions in inflammation—the body's natural response to stress—which can contribute to a host of age-related diseases.

Gratitude journaling isn't merely about feeling good—it's about rewiring your brain to focus on the positive. Regularly jotting down things you're grateful for can enhance your mood, decrease instances of disease, and improve sleep quality. It turns the mind away from toxic emotions, such as resentment and jealousy, and fosters a sense of contentment that's closely linked to overall longevity.

Continuing with the theme of reflection, mindfulness extends to the practice of mindful eating. By paying full attention to the experience of eating—savoring each bite, acknowledging the flavors and textures, and listening to our bodies' hunger cues—we can transform a routine activity into an enriching experience that can prevent overeating and promote digestive health.

Another technique for cultivating inner peace and longevity is visualization, where you create a mental image of a calm, peaceful setting or a desired outcome in your life. It's like a mental rehearsal for relaxation. By envisioning a positive future or a serene environment, you can coax your body into a relaxed state, reducing stress hormones that contribute to aging.

Grounding, also known as 'earthing,' is the practice of connecting with the earth's natural electric charge by walking barefoot on grass, sand, or soil. This may sound esoteric, but emerging studies suggest that this contact can help reduce inflammation and cortisol levels, providing a unique and refreshing path to inner peace.

One cannot overstate the importance of sleep in the pursuit of inner peace and longevity. While we've discussed sleep in the context of physical health, it's equally vital for mental well-being. Insufficient sleep is linked to mood disorders, decreased cognitive function, and even a weakened immune system. Establishing a calming bedtime routine and creating an optimal sleep environment can dramatically impact the quality of our golden years.

When we talk about inner peace, we must also talk about forgiveness—letting go of grudges and bitterness. Harboring these negative emotions can lead to chronic stress, damaging our health and accelerating aging. By practicing forgiveness, we can release these toxic ties to the past and pave the way for a healthier, longer life.

Engaging in regular social activities can also be a form of inner peace cultivation. Strong social ties contribute to a sense of belonging and purpose, factors that can protect against mental decline and improve lifespan. Whether it's volunteering, joining a club, or simply maintaining close relationships, social connectivity is a cornerstone of a well-rounded strategy for longevity.

Developing a hobby or a passion project can inject joy and fulfillment into our lives. Dedicating time to activities we love isn't frivolous—it's essential for mental well-being. The state of 'flow,' where we lose ourselves in an activity, can help mitigate stress and lead to a more profound sense of inner peace.

A less discussed but critical practice is establishing a routine. Regularity and predictability can reduce anxiety and provide a sense of control amidst the chaos of life. A daily routine that includes time for self-care and relaxation can help foster long-term comfort and well-being.

Lastly, embracing a philosophy of lifelong learning can keep our minds nimble and engaged. Challenging ourselves to learn new skills, whether it's a new language or a musical instrument, can combat mental stagnation and promote a youthful outlook on life, which, as we've learned, is instrumental in the aging process.

In summing up these techniques, remember that the pursuit of inner peace is an individual journey. What works for one person may not resonate with another, but the key is consistent practice and finding what aligns with your nature. These methods don't just promise a tranquil mind; they're active contributors to a long and thriving life. As we move forward, let's keep in mind that inner harmony is foundational to our goal of aging not just with grace but with vitality.

Integrating Mindfulness into Daily Life Seamlessly weaving mindfulness into the fabric of our daily existence can be a transformative practice, particularly as we navigate the complex terrain of aging. Rather than relegating mindfulness to a quiet corner of our day, let's explore bringing this powerful ally along for the entire ride.

Mindfulness, the art of being fully present and engaged in the moment without judgment, offers numerous benefits for our mental and physical well-being, especially as we grow older. With regular incorporation into our daily routines, it can enhance awareness, decrease stress, and promote a deep-seated sense of peace that contributes to longevity.

Starting the day with intention sets the tone for mindful living. Upon waking, take a few deep breaths, sensing the life force within you. This simple act can ground you and remind you of the gift of another day. You don't need to carve out a separate time for this; let it be part of the natural process of rising.

As you go about your morning rituals—be it brushing your teeth or making your bed—bring attention to the senses. Notice the texture of the toothbrush, the foamy sensation of the paste, the rhythmic movements. Such tasks become meditative and lose their mundanity when performed with mindfulness.

Breakfast is another opportunity. Rather than mindlessly eating while scrolling through your phone, take a moment to observe your food, appreciating its colors and aroma before savoring each bite.

You're not just nourishing your body; you're also cultivating an attentive spirit.

The daily commute, often a source of tension, can convert into a period of reflection. If you're driving, observe the sensation of the wheel under your hands, the patterns of traffic, and the changing landscape. If you're a passenger, this time can be a sanctuary for mindfulness meditation or simply a chance to gaze out of the window, fully absorbed in the present.

Work demands focus, and mindfulness enhances this. Each task, from answering emails to engaging in meetings, can be approached with a full presence that not only improves performance but also makes the day more enjoyable. When your mind wanders to the past or the future, gently guide it back to now.

Lunchtime is often rushed, but it doesn't have to be. Even a short, mindful pause can reset your system. Taking a brief walk, feeling the sun or the breeze on your skin, and breathing deeply can reconnect you with the here and now.

We know that exercise is key for longevity, and mindfulness converts physical activity from routine to ritual. Mindful walking, or focusing on the body's movements during yoga or weightlifting, enhances the connection between mind, body, and breath. This awareness can make exercise more effective and enjoyable.

Even the after-work unwind time can incorporate mindfulness. Listening fully to a piece of music, engaging in a craft, or simply sitting quietly can be a mindful respite from the day's hustle.

Culinary efforts at dinner can be a time to be fully engaged with the process of creating nourishment. Instead of hurriedly throwing ingredients together, measure each spice mindfully, stir with care, taste with attention, and you'll find that the food isn't the only thing that's been enriched.

Nighttime rituals also offer a prime time for mindfulness. Whether it's skin-care or teeth cleaning, slow down and appreciate each action, each sensation. Allow the day's events to pass through your mind with a nonjudgmental acceptance, preparing you for a restful sleep.

If you find your mind racing as you lie in bed, practice a body scan meditation. Start at your toes and work your way up, sending each part of your body a silent "goodnight." It's a way of telling the body and mind it's time to power down for the day.

In these snippets of daily life, the practice of mindfulness, sometimes subtle, has a cumulative impact. It's like a gentle but persistent wind shaping the landscape of our minds, carving out grooves of peace and resilience that serve us well as we age.

And while the immediate aim is to bring a mindful awareness to everyday activities, the long game here is about fostering a sense of centeredness that carries us gracefully through our years. It's about cultivating an inner sanctuary that can weather the external storms, easing the toll they take on our bodies and spirits.

It's about getting in the driver's seat of our own aging process by taking charge of our moment-to-moment experience. So let mindfulness seep into your day-to-day life, let it be like that favorite melody that hums quietly in the background, and let it guide you towards a life that is lived fully—every single second of it.

Chapter 18:
Financial Health and Longevity

As we've delved into a wealth of strategies for maintaining our physical and mental vigor, let's not overlook the pivotal role of financial well-being in our longevity equation. Think of your finances as the fuel in your longevity tank; without it, even the smoothest-running engine won't get you far. Smart financial planning isn't about hoarding gold for a rainy day—it's about ensuring that your wealth works hand in hand with your health. Every dollar you save and invest wisely is a dollar that you can spend towards sustaining and enhancing the quality of life you've worked so hard to achieve. Financial stress can be a silent ager, corroding your well-being like rust on iron, so embracing sound money habits and longevity-focused financial planning becomes a master key to unlocking a life of sustained health and happiness. As we explore the Nexus of finance and longevity, bear in mind that the seeds you plant today in your financial garden can grow into a lush canopy of security, peace of mind, and enduring well-being. Taking the reins of your financial health means you're not just planning for a future; you're fortifying your present, ensuring that every step you take towards aging gracefully is taken with confidence.

Planning for a Future of Wellness As we traverse through the chapters of this narrative on evergreen vitality, we've digested a smorgasbord of tactics to slow the ticking of our biological clocks. From the alchemy of nutrients that fight the wear of time to the rejuvenation found in sleep's silent sanctuary, the mosaic of longevity is intricate and intensely personal. And now, we pivot to financial health, an oft-understated but pivotal cornerstone of our wellness architecture.

Consider financial health as more than mere numbers on a ledger; it is the sustenance for peace of mind and the fuel for choices that can enrich our lives. Just picture it: financial stability paves the way for stress reduction, access to health-promoting goods and services, and even the luxury of picking organic ingredients over processed foods—all without the specter of monetary worry casting a shadow over our golden years.

But where does one start in this daunting realm of numbers, plans, and investments? It's often said that the best time to plant a tree was twenty years ago; the second best time is now. So, let's cultivate our financial orchard today for a harvest of health down the line. Building a nest egg doesn't necessarily demand being a Wall Street guru; instead, it calls for the adoption of smart, consistent money habits.

Creating a budget is the cornerstone of fiscal prudence. To start, align your spending with your values; does each expense nurture your long-term vitality? Think preventative healthcare checkups, a fitness membership, or maybe a meditation app subscription—all investments in your continuing wellness.

Next, optimizing retirement plans—IRAs, 401(k)s, pensions—assures that when work becomes a choice rather than a necessity, you can make that choice freely. If these terms sound foreign, fret not. Approachable resources abound to demystify these vessels for your savings, ensuring they are not some arcane elixir but a simple tonic for future health.

And lest we forget insurance—it's not just a policy, it's a bulwark against health disruptors that could erode your well-being. Consider long-term care insurance, a potent ally in safeguarding both your funds and future health needs. By addressing potential care costs now, you're architecting a fortification that ensures wellness remains uncompromised.

Of course, it's easy to preach austerity, but depriving oneself isn't the zenith of financial wisdom. Rather, thoughtful spending—aligning your monetary outflow with enriching experiences and self-development—produces a tapestry of events that collectively buffer against the weathering effects of age.

Economic autonomy also enables us to take calculated risks, like changing careers to pursue passion over paycheck or relocating for a lifestyle better suited for longevity. These options are not flights of fancy, but genuine choices when bankrolled by savings that serve as a safety net.

Dare to diversify investments like a carefully assembled dinner plate, balanced with portions of stocks, bonds, and real estate. The variance buffers against market tumult and curates a portfolio as robust and resilient as a well-attended-to body.

Certainly, money can't buy youth, but it can invest in continuance and quality. The judicious use of resources for health checks, state-of-the-art treatments, or even supplements ensures you stay at the crest of the wellness wave. To be clear, this is not embracing indulgence but advocating planning and precision that wages proactive combat against aging's inevitable assault.

Financial literacy isn't just a luxury—it's becoming increasingly essential. It's a narrative that unfolds over a lifetime, and the earlier you become fluent, the more profound the impact on your well-being. Educational workshops, books, even free online content can enlighten pathways previously shrouded in obscurity.

Charitable giving, often overlooked, can also enrich your emotional and spiritual domains. Whether aiding medical research or supporting local health initiatives, philanthropy is the currency of well-being, fostering a sense of connection and purpose that engenders a warm, internal glow that no anti-aging cream can replicate.

And in our journey, it's critical to avoid seduction by quick financial fixes and fads. Much like health, wealth isn't typically spawned from shortcuts. It's cultivated through patience, discipline, and occasionally saying no to immediate pleasures for enduring prosperity.

Finally, as we look down the road, estate planning is equivalent to prepping your physical vessel for its voyage towards the horizon. Wills, health care proxies, and power of attorney documents may seem somber, but they're really affirmations of life—a testament to your wishes and care for those you love, ensuring that your wellness values outlive even yourself.

So there it is—a blueprint for fiscal fitness to complement the body's boundless pursuit of health. As we close this chapter, remember the confluence of money and well-being is not about wealth for wealth's sake. It's about the freedom and ability to make lifestyle choices that uphold and elevate our health for an entire lifespan that not only lasts but thrives with boundless energy and joyous vigor.

Smart Money Habits for Sustained Health As we pivot our attention towards financial well-being in the golden years, we uncover yet another cornerstone to mastering the art of aging gracefully. Let's engage in a conversation about money—not merely in the context of wealth accumulation but through the lens of supporting a sustained, vibrant lifestyle. At its core, financial health isn't about hoarding piles of cash; rather, it's about thoughtful stewardship of resources to ensure that every penny spent is a deliberate investment in your long-term health.

Imagine for a moment a banking system within your body, where every nutritional choice you make is a deposit or a withdrawal from your health account. Similarly, think of your financial habits as the metaphorical equivalents that affect your physical well-being. The analogy isn't far-fetched. Crucial to understanding this symbiosis is recognizing the role that sound financial habits play in removing barriers to a healthy lifestyle and further in accessing cutting-edge healthcare as you age.

First, establish a saving regimen. It sounds basic, right? But, the reality is, saving isn't about setting aside enormous sums—it's the regularity that counts. An incremental approach to saving can create a safety net that acts as a buffer for unforeseen health expenses, the kind not covered by typical insurance plans. A little stash set aside for an unplanned pilates class or a supplemental nutrition program can have a tangible impact on your health trajectory.

Next, educate yourself on health insurance options. As we age, medical care becomes increasingly complex and potentially expensive. Understanding your coverage options and the differences between Medicare, supplemental plans, or long-term care insurance is crucial. Armed with knowledge, you're better positioned to make choices that serve your health needs without draining your finances.

Investing in high-quality, nutrient-dense foods is another form of smart spending. Organic produce and grass-fed meats may come with a higher price tag, but they're packed with the essentials your body craves for repair and resilience. Think of these choices as preemptive strikes against the need for medical interventions down the line.

Consider the financial impact of your home environment. A household less reliant on convenience foods and more focused on sustainable living practices ultimately cultivates a space where health can thrive. Energy-efficient appliances, for example, save money on utilities, allowing for more funds to be directed towards wellness activities.

Pertinent too is the savvy use of tax-advantaged savings accounts such as HSAs or FSAs, where you can allocate money for medical expenses. Such accounts can be a game-changer. They allow you to set aside pre-tax dollars for everything from doctor's visits to necessary medical equipment, hence reducing your taxable income. It's a double win—financial savviness bolstering health readiness.

And let's not gloss over the impact that stress related to financial uncertainty can have on your body. Chronic stress is an age accelerator. Hence, investments in financial planning services or tools that help you track and manage your budget can be invaluable. Not only do they keep you informed, but they also reduce the havoc stress can wreak on your system.

Now, how about the role of physical activity? Aligning your financial choices with accessible exercise forms adds a zestful quality to the aging process. Invest in a comfortable pair of walking shoes or a bike instead of an extra gadget. Or, consider a gym membership that doesn't strain your wallet but gives you a place to build community and engage in routine physical activity.

Preventative health screenings, often covered by insurance, are smart to keep up with, as they can catch issues before they become severe. But here's the catch—knowing when and what screenings are necessary for your age and risk factors takes a bit of research, which pertains to financial literacy as much as it does to health awareness.

On top of these, for those who are able to, investing in preventative healthcare technologies and services — like genomic testing or telemedicine — might sound like a luxury, but they can also be cost-effective in the long run. Emerging healthcare technologies can enable early detection and proactive management of potential health issues, saving not just money but also preserving quality of life.

As we touch on the notion of cost-effectiveness, let us not forget the prescriptions you fill. Generic medications, when available, are a financially astute alternative to brand-name drugs. They contain the same active ingredients and undergo rigorous testing to ensure they're as effective and safe as their branded counterparts.

Smart money habits extend beyond the present moment. That's where retirement planning intersects with longevity. The funds you allocate now towards your retirement can ensure that you maintain autonomy and choice in how you manage your health needs later. After all, financial independence can contribute significantly to mental health, reducing worries about the future.

Utility isn't just for business. Apply this concept to purchases that impact your health. This might mean prioritizing a comfortable mattress that supports restorative sleep over a new TV. Or choosing to spend money on experiences like cooking classes that enhance your culinary skills and wellbeing, rather than on material possessions with fleeting satisfaction.

Finally, embracing technology to manage your finances can streamline the process and free up more time for health-promoting activities. Financial management apps can help you budget efficiently, ensuring you have the resources for a wholesome lifestyle at your fingertips.

In essence, when we talk about anti-aging, the conversation is incomplete without acknowledging the influence of smart financial habits. These habits are the vessels that can carry us through an extended life with independence, security, and health—not as second thoughts, but as a deliberate blueprint for longevity. Indeed, managing your finances with an eye towards overall well-being is perhaps one of the most impactful longevity strategies you can adopt. It's more than just dollars and cents; it's about crafting a lifestyle where health and wealth aren't mutually exclusive but invariably interwoven.

Chapter 19:
The Anti-Aging Home Environment

Transitioning seamlessly from financial savvy in Chapter 18, we pivot to a place of respite and rejuvenation - our homes. It's not just a shelter but an intimate extension of ourselves that can significantly influence our aging process. In this chapter, we'll unveil the lesser-known secrets to curating an anti-aging haven within the four walls where you spend a substantial slice of life. Let's delve into the transformation of living quarters into longevity-promoting landscapes. We'll explore the subtle art of creating spaces that breathe vitality, be it through the type of furniture that supports your body, the colors that stimulate your mind, natural elements that purify your air, or the very layout that keeps you moving. Imagine a home that doesn't just shelter the physical self but also nurtures a state of wellbeing, harmonizing with the body's natural aging rhythm and possibly even giving the sands of time a run for their money.

Creating a Living Space That Promotes Longevity when we consider our journey towards a long and hearty life, the brick and mortar of our daily existence—our living spaces—take on an exceptional significance. After considering the myriad of strategies to bolster longevity through diet, exercise, and social engagement, it's time to cast a thoughtful glance toward the environments where we spend a lion's share of our waking, and sleeping, hours.

Think for a moment about the sanctuaries we call home. They're more than just shelter or stylishly assembled décor; they're context and canvass for our daily lives. The lighting, the air quality, the ergonomics, even the colors on the walls—these elements, when mindfully combined, can be a hidden trove to reinforce the longevity practices we've previously explored.

Let's start with natural light, a powerful, though often underestimated, contributor to well-being. Abundant daylight syncing with our circadian rhythms encourages healthy sleep patterns, which, as we know, can greatly influence our aging process. Ensuring your home maximizes natural light isn't a luxury, it's a longevity strategy. Consider larger windows or skylights—not just for their aesthetic value, but for their health benefits.

The air we breathe is no less critical. Studies tell us that indoor air quality often lags behind outdoor air, packed with unseen pollutants that can undermine our health. An investment in good ventilation systems or air purifiers can pay health dividends down the line. Indoor plants too, are not merely decorative; they are the lungs of your living space, quietly scrubbing the air you breathe.

Sounds inconsequential, doesn't it, the quality of a chair or the height of a countertop? Yet, the ergonomics of your environment play a subtle but persistent role in your bodily health. Furniture that supports your posture and cabinetry that doesn't require a daily stretch or stoop can keep joint pain at bay and maintain mobility as the years roll on. Design your space with an eye to the future, anticipating the comfort and ease you'll want in the years to come.

What's underfoot matters as well. Flooring that mitigates impact and reduces the risk of falls—think cork or rubber—can be a prudent choice, especially as we age. A poorly chosen rug or slippery tile isn't just an aesthetic miscalculation; it can be a hazard to your long-term health. In the same vein, consider your home's navigation: clear paths, good lighting, and minimal clutter are simple corrections that make a tangible difference.

The psychology of color plays a surprising role in our daily mood and, over the long haul, our health. Studies suggest that certain hues can calm the mind or invigorate the spirit. So, painting your space isn't just an act of personal expression, it's a chance to subtly influence your mental health day in and day out. Choose your palette with an aim toward serenity and vitality.

Surround yourself with life. Art that speaks to your soul, photographs that evoke happy memories, even a well-tended aquarium can be sources of daily joy—small affirmations that can collectively stave off the stress that wears on the body over time. These personal touches convert a space from merely functional to deeply nourishing for your spirit—and longevity isn't merely about the body, is it?

As we spend roughly a third of our life sleeping, the bedroom demands a special focus. Beyond a supportive mattress, consider investing in hypoallergenic bedding to reduce the risk of allergens disrupting your sleep. The color choices here too should promote restfulness; soft blues, greens, or creams can create an atmosphere conducive to deep, restorative sleep.

Don't overlook the power of scent. Essential oils diffused through your home can do more than create a pleasant atmosphere; some have properties known to reduce anxiety, improve sleep, or stimulate the mind. Such sensory details craft an environment that leans into the pursuit of longevity with every breath.

A well-appointed kitchen can turn the chore of cooking into a celebration of healthful living. Organize and design your kitchen to make healthy food choices the easiest to access and prepare. Clear counters with space for chopping vegetables, a visible spice rack reminding you of the myriad flavors at your disposal—these nudges toward nutritious meals can bear fruit in long-term health advantages.

Beyond the tangible, it's worth considering the intangible rhythms your home encourages. A dedicated space for meditation or yoga, free from the distractions of daily life, can make committing to these practices easier and more rewarding. When the barriers to mindfulness are removed, consistency—and thus, the benefits—soar.

The practicality of your home layout can also reinforce social connections. Areas conducive to entertaining or simply spaces that make it comfortable for friends to pop in for coffee can foster those vital interpersonal connections that we've learned hold significant sway over our longevity.

Finally, consider your home's ability to adapt to your changing needs over time. Universal design principles—like lever door handles that are easier on the hands or walk-in showers that reduce fall risk—can make your home a haven for aging gracefully. Planning with foresight can ensure that the space that serves you well now will continue to do so in the decades to come.

Every corner of your living space offers an opportunity to support a life rich with vitality and years. As we've shaped our habits in nutrition, exercise, and rest, let's shape our homes with equal intentionality. Our living spaces align with our desire for longevity when every detail is considered not just for its immediate comfort or beauty, but for its nurturing embrace on our longer, fuller lives.

In the panoramic view of the strategies that pave the way to a vibrant old age, the setting in which we carry out our daily dance with time plays a starring role. Let's ensure it's tailored not just to our present comfort, but to a future of sustained wellness. For it's within these very walls we have the honor of crafting a long, joyous, and healthy journey through life.

The Impact of Toxins and How to Minimize Exposure The modern world is replete with conveniences designed to make our lives more comfortable and efficient. However, there's an often unseen trade-off in this equation—exposure to a multitude of environmental toxins. From the air we breathe to the water we drink, the threat lingers, potentially accelerating aging and impeding our pursuit of longevity.

Let's unpack the term 'toxins'. Essentially, these are substances deemed poisonous or potentially harmful to our body, and guess what? They're just about everywhere—from household cleaners to the food supply chain. Here, we'll navigate the labyrinth of where these potential dangers lie and discuss strategies to lessen their impact on our bodies and ultimately, our health span.

Take air pollution, for instance. It's a cocktail of particulate matter, gases, and chemicals that, over time, can wreak havoc on our respiratory and cardiovascular systems. Studies even suggest a link between polluted air and cognitive decline. Prioritizing living situations with good air quality and investing in air purifiers can be game changers.

Water sources aren't immune to toxic infiltration, often containing contaminants that range from heavy metals to pesticides. Ensure your drinking water is clean by using filters that remove these contaminants. And it's not just about what you drink—think of the chemicals potentially seeping through your skin during a hot shower. A filter for your showerhead isn't a luxury; it's a protective layer.

The food we eat can be a highway for toxins directly into our bodies. Pesticides, hormones, and antibiotics are commonly used in agriculture, while processed foods are laden with preservatives and artificial additives. Opt for organic produce when possible, and lean on whole foods over their processed counterparts.

It's not just ingestion; our skin—the body's largest organ—is another absorption site for harmful substances. Skincare and beauty products can harbor phthalates, parabens, and synthetic fragrances that some evidence suggests might disrupt our endocrine systems. Consider sourcing natural and non-toxic personal care items. The philosophy here is simple: if you wouldn't put it in your body, perhaps rethink putting it on your body.

Household cleaners, too, are rife with chemicals that can cause chronic health issues. Think about it—those strong fumes that signal 'clean' are often warning signs of toxic presence. Invest in green, natural cleaning products or produce your own with ingredients like vinegar, baking soda, and essential oils.

Technology, while making our lives easier, also emits pollutants like electromagnetic fields (EMFs). These can cause biological stress, and while the debate on their effects continues, adopting habits like unplugging appliances when not in use and using EMF shields can minimize risk.

Plastic containers are perpetual villains in the toxin tale. BPA (bisphenol A), found in many plastics, is notorious for its potential hormonal effects. Shift towards glass or other non-toxic materials for food storage and reheating.

These adjustments in lifestyle might seem overwhelming, but remember, it's a journey. Start with the low-hanging fruit—improve your diet or change the products you use daily. Every little action is a step toward mitigating the onslaught of environmental aggressors.

Dental amalgam, used in fillings, contains mercury—a potent neurotoxin. If you're getting dental work, inquire about mercury-free alternatives. Similar vigilance is needed in choosing your cookware; non-stick surfaces might make cleanup a breeze, but could off-gas harmful chemicals at high temperatures. Opt for safer cookware like cast iron, stainless steel, or ceramic.

Connection to nature might offer another layer of defense. Plants have a natural ability to absorb and neutralize certain toxins. Develop a green thumb; a home with well-placed houseplants can benefit from nature's own detoxifiers.

Knowledge is power; being informed about potential toxin exposure from various sources enables you to make choices to protect your personal environment. As we push the boundaries of healthy aging, creating a toxin-aware lifestyle is integral to our longevity toolkit.

Never skip the small print. Be it grocery shopping or choosing a new hair dye, scrutinize labels for hidden nasties. Look out for certifications and seals indicating a product is free from common harmful chemicals.

Moving forward, intersperse these detoxifying habits throughout your routines and don't be disheartened if it feels incremental. Each small, sustained practice collectively contributes towards a significant reduction in toxin exposure.

Lastly, remember that our bodies are remarkably resilient and adaptable—if we give them less to fight against toxin-wise, they can focus more on regeneration and repair. Cleaning up our act, quite literally, ushers in a clearer path to a vibrant and youthful existence. With each conscious choice, we're telling our biology and the passage of time that we're not passive participants but active architects of our longevity story.

Chapter 20:
Travel and Leisure for a Younger You

Moving forward from the anti-aging sanctity of our homes, let's expand our horizons to the rejuvenating power of travel and leisure. Just as a sculptor shapes clay into a masterpiece, our experiences mold and invigorate our spirits. Journeying beyond familiar perimeters doesn't just break the monotony; it can add years to our lives and life to our years. Envision the glee in sharing stories of a sun-drenched escapade or the tranquility of a mountain retreat—these aren't just postcards for the mantel, but investments in our youthful essence. Regular getaways are like hitting the refresh button on our biological browsers, they declutter the mind and foster cellular jubilee. Embracing new sights and cultures pumps vitality into our veins and stirs the cognitive cocktail for a sharper, more spirited self. So whether it's discovering a hidden grove or relishing in the cacophony of a bustling city market, we engage in a symphony of experiences that compel our biological clock to sway in youthful rhythm. Don't merely sightsee, live see—each destination is a chapter in the narrative of a younger you.

Incorporating Adventure into a Long Life isn't just about the thrill of exploration or ticking off destinations from a bucket list; it's about weaving a fabric of experiences that keep the senses sharpened, the mind active, and the spirit engaged. In the pursuit of longevity, embracing adventure can be one of the most rewarding aspects, but it requires a shift in perspective.

At the heart of this concept lies the balance between comfort and challenge. Our daily routines provide security, but it's in the novel and unfamiliar that we find growth. Science shows us that stepping out of our comfort zones leads to mental and emotional agility. Consider this: when was the last time you did something for the first time?

New experiences have an uncanny ability to imprint more vividly in our memory, giving us the sense of a life richly lived. Psychological studies indicate that individuals who regularly engage in diverse and novel activities report greater satisfaction. It's not about risky undertakings but about finding joy in the small adventures that life offers.

For one, travel broadens the mind. It's not necessary to journey across the globe, although that is splendid when possible. Even local explorations can offer a fresh perspective. It's about the art of seeing the extraordinary in the ordinary. Take a different route, visit a new park, or dine at an unfamiliar restaurant. Invigorate your senses with fresh sights, sounds, and tastes.

Include learning as part of your adventure. Endeavor to pick up a new language, delve into pottery, or dance lessons. When we learn, we grow, and growth is at the core of staying young at heart. Developing new skills can be particularly potent in maintaining cognitive health as we age, building and strengthening neural pathways that keep the brain resilient.

Getting physical outdoors is also a vital piece of the puzzle. Whether it's hiking, cycling, swimming, or even walking in nature, such activities not only improve physical health but also expose us to new stimuli and environments. There's a profound simplicity in the connection with nature that speaks to the very essence of our being and enlivens us.

Don't allow age to define your capacity for adventure. Remember, it's not merely about physical endurance or extreme sports; it's about allowing yourself to experience wonder and curiosity, just as we naturally did as children. Adapt your adventures to suit your physical abilities, whether it involves gentle walks, gardening, birdwatching, or sailing.

Volunteering can be an adventure of the heart. Giving your time to a cause can propel you into new communities, challenge your perspectives, and fill you with a sense of purpose. Such endeavors remind us that life's value is not just measured in years, but in the richness of experiences we share with others.

Embrace technology to turn ordinary days into adventures. Virtual reality can transport you to foreign lands or historical moments, a testament to humanity's inventiveness. You might not be physically there, but it expands your horizons all the same.

Mind-set is another piece of the adventure puzzle. Viewing the aging process as a journey rather than a decline opens up new doors of possibilities. See each year as an invitation to experience something different rather than a step away from youth.

Despite all these suggestions, one mustn't forget the element of spontaneity. Sometimes, the greatest adventures are unplanned. Allow yourself to be flexible, to welcome the unexpected, and to revel in the joy of serendipitous discoveries. After all, it's those surprise moments that often become the most treasured memories.

Prioritize your adventures by turning them into non-negotiable aspects of your life. Just as you would not skip a doctor's appointment, schedule regular 'adventure days.' By doing so, you're committing to continually experiencing life to the fullest, which in turn bolsters your mental and physical health.

Of course, adventures can also be shared — another longevity secret. Social connections boost our mental health, and what better way to bond with loved ones than through shared experiences? Whether it's with a partner, friend, or a group with similar interests, together you create stories that last a lifetime.

If concerns about safety and health are holding you back, plan wisely. Research destinations, prepare adequate supplies, know your medical needs, and don't be shy to ask for assistance if necessary. Adventure doesn't have to be risky to be rewarding.

To sum up, incorporating adventure into a long life isn't a diversion from the serious business of staying healthy; it's an essential component of it. It keeps the heart young, the mind nimble, and the spirit soaring. So, go on, build your own tapestry of adventures. After all, life isn't just about the number of breaths we take, but about the moments that take our breath away.

The Health Benefits of Regular Vacations Grab those sunglasses and prepare to dive into the rejuvenating world of regular vacations. You've probably heard countless times that taking time off is good for the soul, but have you ever considered the tangible health benefits it brings, particularly in the context of aging? Each trip we embark on is not just an escape from the daily grind, but also a leap toward longevity and enhanced vitality.

Let's start with stress, the not-so-silent saboteur of health and well-being. Work deadlines, family obligations, and the persistent pinging from our smartphones all contribute to our stress levels. Vacations interrupt this relentless onslaught, offering a reprieve that is both necessary and invigorating. The reduction of stress from stepping away from your daily environment has profound effects, decreasing the risk of heart disease and promoting better mental health—two essential factors in the art of aging gracefully.

Moreover, vacations are linked to improved cardiovascular health. Studies have suggested that those who vacation regularly are less likely to suffer from heart attacks or coronary death compared to those who rarely take time off. It's as though travel puts a pause on the pressures that frequently pummel our hearts, giving our most vital organ a much-needed break.

Imagine this: You're lounging on a sun-drenched beach, waves lapping at the shore, with no agenda other than to relish the moment. Your mind naturally drifts into a state of mindfulness, fully engaged and savoring the here and now. This mindful immersion has ripple effects on mental health. People who vacation frequently report feeling happier and more content with life—not just during the trip, but extending into the weeks that follow. Thus, regular vacations can act as a reset button, lending clarity and reducing symptoms of depression and anxiety.

Musculoskeletal disorders, the aches and pains associated with aging, can also be alleviated by the physical activity that often accompanies travel. Hiking through a national park, swimming in the ocean, or even navigating a new city on foot increases physical activity levels, which are crucial for maintaining muscle mass and bone density as we age.

Sleep, the cornerstone of recovery for our bodies, tends to improve while on vacation. Away from the blue light of screens and the incessant call of responsibilities, many people find that their sleep quality increases. And we know that good sleep is intrinsically linked to a range of health benefits, such as improved memory, reduced inflammation, and better immune function—all allies in the battle against aging.

Engagement with people, cultures, and environments that differ from our normal routine also enriches our brain health. This intellectual stimulation sparks curiosity and promotes neural plasticity, helping to keep aging minds sharp and responsive. It's as though every new experience on vacation lays another brick on the pathway to cognitive resilience.

Exposure to different environments when travelling can also boost your immune system. Being exposed to diverse bacteria and conditions challenges the immune system in a good way, teaching it to be more adaptive and robust—the protective armor we need for a long, invigorating life.

Let's not forget about the joy of anticipation. Planning and looking forward to a vacation can be nearly as beneficial as the trip itself. The psychological lift that comes from expectation can carry one through mundane or challenging times, serving as a beacon of light that promises rest and rejuvenation and encourages a forward-thinking mindset.

Regular vacations can also bolster creativity. Whether it's the tranquil surroundings of a secluded beach or the bustling streets of an urban center that's alive with art and history, stepping outside your routine can lead to bursts of inspiration, novel ideas, and innovative solutions. As we age, continuing to nourish creativity is key to a vibrant and engaging life.

Articulating the value of experiences over material possessions is a conversation that's been gaining ground in recent years, and the rationale is clear when looking at how vacations contribute to long-term happiness. Accumulating memories, rather than things, has a lasting positive effect on our well-being. Hence, as we invest in travel, we're truly investing in a reservoir of joyful reminiscences that can provide sustenance in our later years.

There's also evidence to suggest that regular vacations can increase lifespan. While this may sound too good to be true, consider the cumulative effect of reduced stress, increased physical activity, enhanced sleep, and all the other benefits previously mentioned. When you put it all together, it's easy to see how vacations can add years to your life—and life to your years.

Intertwined with the concept of longevity is the quality of life. As we age, our goal isn't merely to extend our time on this earth but to enhance the richness of our experiences within that time. Vacations provide a unique opportunity to deepen bonds with loved ones, to collect stories that will be recounted for generations, and to foster a sense of connection and belonging in the wider world. These are the intangible threads that weave the fabric of a life well-lived.

Finally, the newfound perspectives gained from regular travel can provide the impetus for positive life changes. Many return from vacations with a renewed vigor to take care of their health, to prioritize what's truly important, or to finally embark on lifestyle changes that have been simmering on the back burner. In this way, vacations can serve as catalysts for holistically rejuvenating one's approach to health and aging.

So, when contemplating your next wellness strategy, make sure to include regular vacations on the list. They're not just a fleeting escape from reality; they are a channel through which we can experience a more youthful, healthier existence. And isn't that what we're all searching for as we navigate the intricacies of aging? Not just more time, but the vitality and zest to make every moment truly count.

Chapter 21:
Fashion and Identity

As we've cruised through various facets of aging, it's clear how integral lifestyle choices are to staying vibrantly young at heart. Now, we approach an often underestimated aspect—fashion. Consider it less about superficiality and more a celebration of personal identity. It's intriguing how our wardrobe choices reflect and influence our self-perception. By embracing fashion as a medium of self-expression, we assert our individuality and embrace our creativity, two fundamental components of cognitive vitality. And here's the kicker: Cultivating a sense of style can do wonders for our confidence, which, as you've guessed, is interlaced with our overall wellness. The clothes we don bring more than a pop of color or texture to our daily life; they carry the power to invigorate our spirit and pepper our steps with an extra dose of confidence. Simply put, the way we dress can be a dynamic, silent language that speaks volumes about who we are, who we aspire to be, and how we navigate the world around us as we age.

Dressing for Vitality and Confidence As we journey through the chapters of health and wellness, considering the fabric that wraps our very skin seems all too fitting. Turning a fresh page, we'll dive into how the subtleties of one's attire can not only reflect their spirit but actually shape it. Imagine the clothes you wear as a conversation; while they might initially serve to communicate to others, they also speak volumes to you about you. Your choice of garb can invigorate you with vitality and swathe you in the armor of self-assurance.

Let's ponder the way colors infuse energy into our beings. Picture the radiance of a crimson dress or the serenity of a sky-blue shirt. These aren't mere pigments; they're psychological tools at your disposal. The shades and tones you choose can lift your spirit and command the energy you emit and absorb throughout the day. Have you ever noticed feeling a bit perkier when dressed in a bright color? That's no accident; it's the interplay of aesthetics and neurology—grabbing a palette of hues when you dress could be your first step towards a zestful presence.

Material matters matter. It might sound trite but bear with me. The tactile sensation of soft cotton, the luxurious caress of silk, or the grounded touch of hemp—these fabrics interact with our skin, the body's largest organ. We mustn't dismiss the influence of a comfortable outfit on our mood and poise. Aligning comfort with style isn't just practical; it's a form of self-respect that communicates to the world and ourselves that we are worth the best.

How about the cut and form of our wardrobe selections? The flow of a maxi dress, the structure of a well-tailored suit—they offer more than aesthetic appeal. They influence our posture, our body language, and even the way we walk through a room. Slipping into an outfit that compliments your body's landscape is akin to embracing your physical form with confidence, which, as we've learned, can have astounding effects on longevity and vitality.

Here's a thought: accessorizing isn't just about embellishment. Choosing the right accessories can transform an outfit, of course, but it also enhances our ability to express our individuality. A bold necklace or a classic watch is a proclamation of identity. Every accessory tells a story, ours, which contributes to a deeper sense of self and, in turn, bolsters our confidence.

Let's not sidestep the subject of shoes. They are, quite literally, the foundation of our attire. The importance of supportive, comfortable footwear in maintaining an active lifestyle can't be overstated. Yet, there's also a psychological component to consider. The right shoes can empower us, adding a spring to our step and a lift to our spirits, signifying readiness to stride forth into the world with purpose.

Seasonality plays its part, too. We're not just talking about dressing appropriately for the weather—though that's important for comfort and health—but also about aligning with the rhythms of nature. Embrace the transformation that each season brings, and let your wardrobe mirror the bloom or fall of the environment around you. It's a way of staying connected to the world, which, as we've gathered in previous chapters, is integral to our well-being.

Now, the importance of grooming cannot be overstated when we talk about dressing for vitality and confidence. It's not just about the threads but how we present ourselves in them. Neatness and personal style go hand in hand in conveying who we are. Styling one's hair or taking the time for a clean shave can be acts of mindfulness that remind us we are worth the effort, every single day.

Transitioning to sustainability, there's something to be said for knowing the origins of what we wear. Choosing ethically made clothes can provide peace of mind and a sense of contribution to a greater good. It's a subtle yet powerful way to feel connected to your values and demonstrate that you care—not only about your appearance but also about the impact you have on the world.

Quality over quantity is a mantra for many aspects of life, and it rings particularly true for our wardrobes. Investing in fewer pieces that are well-made and timeless not only ensures durability but also creates a connection with our attire. Quality clothing can be like an old friend, growing with us and adapting to our changing lives and bodies—embodying our personal history and evolution.

Fashion and function must find harmony. The garments that grace our bodies should not hinder our movements or our lifestyle. Active wear should facilitate activity, business attire should exude professionalism without constriction, and leisure wear should allow full relaxation. In aligning these elements, we craft a wardrobe that supports rather than suppresses our daily endeavors.

Finally, revisiting the personal element—what sparks joy in you? Marie Kondo may have been onto something with her tidying ethos. If an article of clothing no longer serves you, let it go. By curating a closet that resonates with who you are and who you aim to be, you pave the way to a vibrant image and self.

Consider the act of dressing each day as a ritual. A ritual that isn't just about covering up or showing off, but about deliberate choices that empower your body, fortify your mind, and celebrate the life you live. Your attire is an outward expression of your zest for life, your experiences, and the unique contributions you make to the world. Dress for yourself first, and watch the world respond to your radiance.

Bearing in mind these threads of thought, the unassuming act of choosing our attire emerges as a significant facet of our quest for longevity. It's a testament to the power of everyday actions in shaping our well-being. As we drape ourselves daily, let's do so with the intention of honoring the vitality within, crafting an exterior that both reflects and amplifies the youthful spirit we've so mindfully nurtured.

In closing, remember that vitality and confidence are not only the outcomes but also the catalysts of how we choose to present ourselves to the world. As we continue to unravel the tapestry of strategies for a life full of vitality, let's weave fashion and personal style in as integral pieces of the longevity puzzle. Here, between the warp and weft of fabric, lies the shimmering thread of a vibrant life lived with intention and style.

The Influence of Personal Style on Aging Moving seamlessly from the spectrum of health factors that influence aging, we now enter the realm where the aesthetic meets the scientific—our personal style. Odd as it may seem to connect your wardrobe choices with longevity, the threads we choose to wear stretch beyond the fabric, sewing into our very notion of self and well-being.

Your personal style isn't merely a superficial layer of your identity; it's a conversation between you and the world about who you are—and, importantly, who you are becoming as you age. Walking down this lane, we're not talking solely about fashion but a broader sense of style encompassing attire, grooming, and the individual flair that makes one stand out or blend in. It's about expressing individuality and how that expression influences our perception and experience of aging.

The first stitch in this fabric is confidence. When you are attired in a way that resonates with your sense of self, that alignment can confer a sense of control, empowerment, and positivity. It's common wisdom that when you look good, you feel good, but let's embellish that piece of wisdom with some data. Research suggests that mental well-being can be significantly impacted by how we perceive our physical appearance; it affects our mood, social interactions, and even our posture—all aspects that play vital roles in the way we age.

Diving deeper, think about the messages your personal style sends about age. Subconsciously, your wardrobe choices might reflect cultural narratives about aging—whether you embrace them or resist. Estranging yourself from certain styles 'appropriate' for your age can serve as a powerful reminder that age is but a number, not a strict guideline for self-expression. To wear what you love, regardless of societal expectations, is to practice a form of daily rebellion against ageism.

Furthermore, personal style can be a means of staying engaged with the world. The act of choosing, curating, and wearing clothes can be seen as an ongoing project that keeps one mentally active and socially involved. It's like painting on a canvas that doesn't remain static, it evolves with time—encouraging adaptability, which is a cornerstone for aging gracefully.

When we contemplate the impact of style on physical well-being, let's not overlook comfort. It's not superficial to seek out garments that not only represent who you are but also respect the evolving needs of your body. Well-fitting, comfortable clothing can prevent skin irritation, boost circulation, support mobility, and even regulate body temperature—small factors that cumulatively contribute to healthier aging.

Yet, personal style can also have potential downsides if it becomes a source of stress. The pressure to 'look young' can lead to unhealthy habits, overconsumption, and mental strain—all of which can accelerate the aging process. It's crucial to strike a balance between self-expression and self-acceptance, between striving for an ideal and savoring the beauty of the present.

Consider also the role of grooming and skincare routines as extensions of your personal style. These daily rituals not only help maintain the health and youthfulness of your appearance but can serve meditative and therapeutic roles, promoting relaxation and a sense of self-care that boosts overall well-being.

Grooming rituals and clothing choice also intersect with the idea of routine, a concept that is covered in more depth in other sections of this work. A consistent routine in dressing and self-care reinforces structure in one's life—providing small, but powerful, anchors as life's pace changes with age.

The accessibility of one's style choices is another thread to consider. As we age, simplicity, ease of wear, and maintenance can become increasingly valuable. Clothing that is easy to put on, care for, and maintain can reduce unnecessary hurdles, making daily life smoother and more enjoyable. This isn't to encourage a slide into apathy towards one's appearance but to prompt thoughtful choices that maintain dignity without unnecessary complexity.

Having touched upon the mental and physical, we must not ignore the social aspect. Your style affects not just how you perceive yourself, but how others perceive you. It can influence the quality of your interactions and the strength of your relationships. And as we know from earlier chapters, social connections are a bedrock of longevity. When style helps you connect effectively with others, it contributes positively to your healthspan.

Upcycling your wardrobe is another aspect of personal style that speaks volumes about your approach to aging. Embracing a timeless style, maintaining and repurposing clothing, or adapting garments to fit your evolving body—these are practices that not only demonstrate sustainability but reinforce a narrative where age is met with creativity and resilience.

Lastly, personal style can serve as a conduit for memories and heritage, a means of storytelling that threads through generations. The act of wearing a vintage piece or incorporating a family heirloom into your wardrobe is a connection to your past and a legacy for the future—a subtle admittance that aging is an ongoing conversation with time.

In wrapping up this pattern of thought, it's clear that the influence of personal style on aging is multifaceted and deeply personal. While style choices alone won't dictate one's longevity, they play an intricate role in shaping the daily experience of growing older. They're a statement of being, a personal manifesto projected to the world, and within their folds, they carry the potential to influence health, happiness, and how gracefully one moves through the years.

Now, as we consider the tapestry of influences that contribute to aging well, let us carry forward the understanding that the colors we choose to adorn ourselves with are not frivolous decorations but, in fact, tangible expressions of our individual journey through life.

Chapter 22:
Longevity Around the World

Embarking on a global voyage in our pursuit of longevity, we realize that extended lifespans aren't solely the product of cutting-edge treatments or the latest supplements; instead, they often arise from time-tested wisdom embedded in various cultures. As we explore enclaves where age is merely a number and vitality a way of life, communities otherwise known as the Blue Zones emerge as a fascinating focus. These pockets of the planet offer not just a glimpse into extraordinary lifespans but also practical insights on harmonizing our everyday choices with ancestral truths. Observing their approach to diet, exercise, and community sheds light on the deeply woven tapestry of factors contributing to longevity. Delving into the heart of Sardinia, the serene coasts of Okinawa, and the olive groves of Ikaria, we absorb the cultural essence that nurtures a longer, healthier existence, diverging from a narrow focus on individual habits to embrace a holistic ethos of aging. It's here, in the cross-cultural examination, that we discover the synergy between place, practice, and the profound connection to our world, and how we can adapt these lessons to the canvas of our own lives. By integrating these age-old secrets into our modern existence, the quest for longevity becomes an artful blend of respect for tradition and the embrace of contemporary health principles, guiding us to weave a rich pattern of life that endures through generations.

Lessons from the Blue Zones What if the fountain of youth isn't a mythical spring but a mosaic of lifestyles quietly practiced in pockets of the world known as Blue Zones? These regions boast a disproportionately high number of centenarians and we've got to ask, what's their secret? It's an enthralling suggestion for any health enthusiast: that by mirroring certain lifestyle habits, you might just tap into a blueprint for longevity.

Dan Buettner, a National Geographic Fellow and author, identified these longevity hotspots and gave them the title Blue Zones. They are Sardinia in Italy, Okinawa in Japan, Loma Linda in California, Nicoya in Costa Rica, and Ikaria in Greece. Each of these communities boasts unique cultural norms, yet share common practices that seem to contribute significantly to their residents' long and healthy lives.

One of the cornerstones shared among Blue Zone populations is their diet. Predominantly plant-based, their meals are a colorful ensemble of legumes, whole grains, fruits, vegetables, nuts, and seeds. It's not just about what they eat, but also about how much. Embodying what Okinawans call 'Hara Hachi Bu,' they eat until they're only 80% full, avoiding excessive calorie intake which can be a stressor on the body over time.

Remarkably, movement is woven seamlessly into their daily routine. Instead of carving out dedicated times for exercise, physical activity is a natural byproduct of their lifestyle. Whether it's tending gardens, walking to a neighbor's house, or shepherding livestock, Blue Zone inhabitants unknowingly perform low-intensity physical activity throughout the day, supporting their body's natural functions and contributing to their overall health.

Stress, regrettably, is universal. However, in these zones, a unique relationship to stress emerges. People have cultural strategies to mitigate stress like ancestor veneration in Okinawa, or the daily siesta in Ikaria. Chronic stress has detrimental effects on the body's systems, influencing aging, so these stress-management practices may confer distinct advantages.

A powerful lesson from the Blue Zones is in the value of social connections and maintaining a sense of community. The elder members aren't just included; they're revered. Family and community take priority, offering a support network that not only bolsters psychological well-being but thereby improves physical health, too.

Another central element that threads through the lifestyle of Blue Zones is purpose. Known as 'Ikigai' in Japan and 'Plan de Vida' in Nicoya, this sense of purpose and knowing your role within the community acts as a driving force that keeps individuals active and mentally sharp.

Let's talk about alcohol. Unlike the tendencies of many Western societies, inhabitants of the Blue Zones enjoy alcohol in moderation. Sardinians, for instance, drink Canonau wine, which contains high levels of antioxidants. The key is moderate consumption, regularly but not excessively.

While religious practices vary across the Blue Zones, spirituality and faith seem to be common threads. Participation in spiritual practices has been correlated with lower levels of stress, a sense of belonging, and that all-important community connection.

Blue Zoners tend to wake with the sun and sleep following its descent, aligning their circadian rhythms naturally with the environment. This sleep pattern is not only refreshing but also supports numerous body processes essential for health maintenance and disease prevention.

From observing Blue Zones, one could argue that what they don't consume is equally important as what they do. Highly processed foods, sugars, and artificial additives seldom find their way onto their plates.

Their distances from industrialized food chains may, in fact, be a protective factor in their longevity.

Each of these Blue Zone areas has provided us with a wealth of lessons. It's clear that longevity isn't due to a singular magic bullet, but rather a symphony of lifestyle elements that most importantly can be replicated to some degree no matter where we live. For instance, we can nurture our social relationships, find our purpose, and move naturally through our environment.

The Blue Zones teach us about the importance of balance. From diet and exercise to work and leisure, a harmonious life could indeed be the recipe for a longer, healthier existence. By incorporating aspects of these habits and values into our own lives, we may not guarantee a lifespan of a century, but we could certainly tip the scales in favor of vitality and health.

So, how do we begin? It starts with a choice, a choice to emulate the best practices of these centenarians - not through drastic overhauls, but through incremental, consistent changes that integrate seamlessly into our routines.

Ultimately, the insights gleaned from the Blue Zones aren't merely feel-good stories or unattainable lifestyles. They are real-life testimonies to the power of lifestyle choices in shaping our health and longevity. They invite us to question and, more importantly, to take action. By integrating these age-defying strategies, we can all aspire to not just a longer life but a life brimming with vitality, connection, and purpose.

Cultural Approaches to Anti-Aging After exploring the landscape of nutrition, exercise, and other individual modalities for slowing the aging process, we turn our gaze to the broader panoramas painted by various cultures around the globe. These cultural canvases reveal a plethora of anti-aging approaches that are as diverse as the societies from which they emanate. They form a tapestry weaved with tradition, social habits, and collective values, each strand offering insights into longevity that transcend the boundaries of conventional Western medicine.

Intriguingly, many of these cultural methodologies aren't packaged as anti-aging strategies per se, but rather as a way of life. Take, for instance, the celebrated Mediterranean lifestyle, which beguiles scientists and laypeople alike with its deceptively simple concoction of fresh produce, abundant olive oil, and a penchant for communal dining. Here, "anti-aging" isn't merely a buzzword; it's a delightful consequence of living within a network that cultivates joy, health, and connectedness at every meal.

Similarly, the Japanese practice of "hara hachi bu," which suggests eating until you're 80% full, subtly encourages calorie restriction without the harsh rigidity of diets. It is this gentle philosophy of not pushing the limits, of finding satiety in moderation, that contributes to the impressive longevity observed in regions like Okinawa, where the saying originates.

Equally fascinating is the Scandinavian embrace of nature and the outdoors known as "friluftsliv." By prioritizing time in the open air, regardless of weather conditions, the Nordic populations revere the restorative powers of the natural world. This immersion in nature isn't just for the spirit; it imparts physical benefits like vitamin D from sunlight, and the mental health advantages of being amongst trees and streams.

The concept of "sobremesa" in Spanish-speaking countries is another cultural gem. It's the art of lingering around the table after a meal, conversing with family and friends, savoring the social aspect of dining rather than rushing back to work or personal tasks. This stress-reducing practice encourages mindfulness and fosters strong social ties, both proven to be powerful allies against premature aging.

Across cultures, the importance of a supportive community is a recurring theme. In many African societies, the sense of ubuntu—"I am because we are"—stresses interconnectivity and altruism. This emphasis on social cohesion and mutual care builds resilience against the wear and tear of aging by cultivating a robust social support network that buffers against life's challenges.

Let us not overlook the Indian subcontinent, where the ancient health system of Ayurveda advocates for a personalized approach to longevity. This millennia-old wisdom emphasizes balance among the body, mind, and spirit, and prescribes daily routines involving natural herbs, yoga, and meditation—all cornerstones of a holistic anti-aging regimen that aligns with the modern push for personalized medicine.

Traditional Chinese Medicine (TCM), with its origins lost in antiquity, also focuses on equilibrium—the yin and yang of existence. This balance is considered essential for a long and healthy life. Practices like tai chi and qigong merge gentle movement, breath control, and meditation, improving both physical and mental faculties in a synergy believed to fortify against the ravages of time.

In Latin America, the siesta is a cultural institution often linked to a slower pace of life. While modern lifestyles threaten this tradition, the principle behind it remains valuable. Restorative rest, something we've all but forgotten in our hustle culture, is embraced here as an antidote to stress, with the potential to curtail inflammation and enhance overall wellbeing—key factors in longevity.

Turning to the Middle East, we find the "hammam," or traditional bathhouse, where cleansing the body goes hand in hand with rejuvenating the mind and communal bonding. These bathhouses offer more than just hygiene—they stand as sanctuaries for downtime and self-renewal, which are essential for a balanced approach to slowing down the clock.

Meanwhile, in the villages of Bhutan, the Gross National Happiness index prevails over Gross Domestic Product as a measure of prosperity. This unique approach prioritizes the collective contentment over mere economic output, resulting in a culture where mental well-being is a public affair and a preventive measure against stress-induced aging.

Each of these cultural practices carries an implicit understanding that lifestyle, environment, and community play indispensable roles in the quest for longevity. They invite us to reassess our individualistic focus on the physical aspects of anti-aging and to consider the power of joy, traditions, and relationships in our pursuit of a life well-lived.

And yet, we can't simply transplant these practices wholesale into our lives. Each must be weighed and adapted to our personal situations, our individual sociocultural contexts, and integrated with modern scientific knowledge. How do we reconcile these time-honored traditions with the relentless advance of medical technology and the individualistic tendencies of Western culture? It's a dance of integration, where respect for global wisdom complements cutting-edge science.

As I've traversed these myriad cultural landscapes, gathering wisdom like precious gems along the way, I must emphasize a crucial realization. There is an art to aging gracefully, and it is not one brushed with a single stroke but with a multi-hued palette that considers the whole human experience in its design.

So as we pen the concluding chapters of our own life narratives, it behooves us to paint with the broadest brush, considering not just the lines of our individual choices, but the colors of our cultural milieu. By doing so, we may just find that the secret to a timeless existence has been written in the stories of our collective human journey all along.

Chapter 23:
The Importance of Routine Medical Check-Ups

Now we've traversed the globe, gathered wisdom from centenarians, and tailored our lifestyles for peak vitality, and yet, it's the rigmarole of routine medical check-ups that provides the real linchpin in our quest for longevity. Woven into the fabric of our health-conscious tapestry, these check-ups are more than mere calendar reminders – they're our personal reconnaissance missions on the battleground against aging. Imagine the human body as a sophisticated piece of machinery, with these check-ups serving as critical maintenance to ensure every component operates smoothly. By staying ahead of potential health snags, catching the whispers of discordant cells or the early murmurs of a once-silent heart issue, we can recalibrate our well-being in real-time. The check-ups are not just about prevention; they're about empowerment – equipping you with the information you need to make informed decisions about your health. In this chapter, let's delve into how these medical rendezvous can be the checkpoints on your journey to an enduring and robust existence, and remember that while aging is inevitable, informed aging is a choice.

Key Screenings and Tests for Long-Term Health So, you're invested in the long game of health — the smart play. Taking care of yourself today is like planting seeds for a lush garden you can enjoy further down the path. Simple, right? But how do we keep an eye on our health's horizon? Enter the realm of screenings and tests, crucial checkpoints along our journey.

First off, our heart is the indefatigable engine of our lives, beating away from the cradle to the golden years. Cardiovascular health screenings should be on your regular checklist. This includes blood pressure measurements, cholesterol levels, and a heart rate check-up. Do you know your numbers? They're not just figures; they're signposts pointing you towards longevity or cautioning you of bumps ahead.

Next up, cancer screenings — a subject that can make many wince. But early detection stands as our most robust defense. Women, remember to schedule your mammograms and Pap smears. Men, don't sidestep the PSA test and any other prostate health evaluations. And for everyone's shared script, colonoscopies should be headliners from the age of 45 or earlier if your family history cues an earlier curtain rise.

Bone density scans might not make your headlines now, but fast-forward a few seasons — trust me, they'll be trending in your health newsfeed. Osteoporosis is sneaky. It tiptoes silently until — snap — a fracture tattles on it. Women, you're in the spotlight post-menopause, but men, this is not a one-act play; osteoporosis can be your drama, too.

Let's touch upon diabetes. This modern scourge masquerades as a mere inconvenience until the mask falls and reveals dire consequences for heart, sight, and extremities. A simple blood sugar level test, maybe an HbA1c, can unfold your glucose narrative. Don't like needles? Consider this a quick prick for a wealth of insight.

Concerned about liver and kidney function? You should be. These backstage workers deserve their health spotlight. Regular blood tests can provide a peep behind the curtain to ensure these organs are hitting all their cues without fluffing their lines.

Speaking of blood, let's chat about the liquid life force coursing through our veins. Blood tests can profile a library of wellness information. Got enough iron? How's the thyroid doing its hormonal ballet? These aren't just advisable; they're chapters of your health anthology waiting to be read.

Thyroid function tests shouldn't be overshadowed here. An over- or underactive thyroid can mimic or magnify aging symptoms. Getting this checked is like tuning your body's thermostat to the right temperature for optimal living.

Vision and hearing tests — some might shrug these off until the world becomes muffled or blurred. Routine checks can catch glaucoma, cataracts, or the slow recession of auditory sharpness. Why not keep the symphony of life in high fidelity and the panorama clear as long as possible?

With our longevity treasure map unfolding, dentistry checks mustn't be overlooked treasure chest. Gum disease links to heart disease, diabetes, and even certain cancers. Biannual dental check-ups? Consider them a trusty compass to guide you through the fog of future health challenges.

Amidst this itinerary of screening travels, take a detour into your personal biosphere — genetic screenings. They're not just for ancestry enthusiasts. They can alert you to predispositions, giving you a head start in the race against potential health adversities.

The ladies' exclusive — ovarian and breast cancer genetic screenings — BRCA genes. Tailor your screening schedule based on these results; it's like having a bespoke map for the health journey ahead.

And gentlemen, it's not just about community shared screenings. Prostate and testicular exams are often whispered about but shout it out loud — they're lifesavers. Figuratively and literally.

Age brings wisdom, they say, and with wisdom comes vaccinations. These aren't just for the young — shingles, pneumococcal pneumonia, and the flu are a few guest stars that aging immune systems become susceptible to. Keep up with immunizations, because prevention is still the best script we have in the anti-aging playbook.

Lastly, it's essential to recognize your skin as the protagonist it is — the largest organ, in fact. Regular skin checks for new or changing spots or moles can be the most straightforward scene in your health narrative. Yet, it can dramatically alter the plot if melanoma enters stage left.

Remember, these screenings and tests are not just appointments. They are investments — personal stakes placed in the fertile ground of tomorrow's wellness. So, knit them into the fabric of your life's routine, ensuring the longevity you're aspiring to is not just a hope but a well-charted destiny.

Navigating the Healthcare System As we entwine the intricate threads of aging and well-being, an important piece of fabric requiring keen attention is the healthcare system. It's no secret that as we journey through time's relentless march, more frequent encounters with various healthcare professionals become a fact of life. To seamlessly navigate this intricate maze, it's essential to become a savvy healthcare consumer – proactive, informed, and strategic in managing your health partnerships.

Start by understanding your health insurance coverage inside and out. This is the roadmap that guides which turns you can take and which roads are perhaps less traveled due to coverage constraints. Knowing your policy not only empowers you with choice but can also shield you from unexpected out-of-pocket expenses that, let's be honest, no one is ever excited to encounter.

Establishing a strong primary care relationship is like building a lighthouse in the fog. This healthcare professional becomes your guide, helping you make sense of complex information, directing you to the right specialists, and tracking your overall health. They're the custodians of your medical history, and in many ways, your first defense when it comes to anti-aging strategies.

When referrals are on the table, quality and compatibility with specialists are paramount. It's about more than just accepting your insurance; it's about finding experts who align with your approach to aging and wellness. They should be partners in your journey, open to discussing everything from traditional treatments to innovative alternatives that could give you an edge in managing aging.

Many people find the prescription management process to be a convoluted affair. Be proactive. Ask your pharmacist questions about drug interactions, particularly as your medication list expands. They are a treasure trove of information and can help you steer clear of unwanted side effects that could slow you down.

Health records have gone digital, and there's incredible value in staying up-to-date with this technology. Online patient portals are your secret weapon, granting you immediate access to your medical information, easing communication with your healthcare team, and simplifying appointment scheduling.

The value of preventive care can't be overstated. These are the scheduled maintenance intervals for your body, detecting issues early, when they're most amenable to treatment. Engage actively in your screenings and immunizations; they are key pieces in the longevity puzzle.

Tackling healthcare costs can be as complex as the care itself. Learn about available financial assistance programs if needed; there's no point in adding financial stress to the preexisting complexities of managing health, as we know stress is a notorious ager.

There's an undeniable link between healthcare providers' bedside manner and patient outcomes. You deserve a healthcare team that listens, empathizes, and communicates clearly. If you're not being heard or respected, it's more than okay to seek a provider who values your perspective as much as you do.

Remember, managing chronic conditions effectively is crucial in slowing aging. A healthcare system that's geared toward chronic disease management can be especially beneficial. Look for programs or providers who not only treat but also educate and empower you to take control of your condition.

Keep an eye out for healthcare innovations. The field of anti-aging medicine is dynamic, and new treatments and technologies emerge at a rapid pace. Stay informed and ask your provider about the potential benefits (and risks) of the latest therapies that may boost your longevity.

As life progresses, so does the need for specialized care. Geriatricians are doctors who specialize in the care of the aging population. They understand the nuances of aging physiology and can tailor your care plan to help you maintain vitality for as long as possible.

Building a network of support within the healthcare system can seem daunting, but remember that patient advocacy groups and navigators exist to help you. They can provide guidance, support, and assistance when facing the more bewildering aspects of the system.

Health literacy is your shield as you traverse the healthcare battlegrounds. It's imperative to educate yourself about your conditions and potential treatments. Misinformation can lead you down perilous paths, so always discuss information you've read or heard with your healthcare provider.

In conclusion, recognize that you're the captain of your own health ship. While the seas of the healthcare system might get rough, with a compass of knowledge and a crew of dependable health professionals, you can set sail towards a horizon of longevity with confidence and grace.

Let's acknowledge that our bodies are akin to complex ecosystems, and maintaining them requires diligent, informed cooperation with our healthcare environment. It's about fitting the pieces together in a manner that serves our long-term vitality, allowing us to experience life's rich tapestry for as long – and as fully – as possible.

Chapter 24:
Preparing for a Graceful Transition

We've journeyed through a wealth of tactics to sustain our vitality, but let's pivot to embrace the quieter, often unspoken realities of aging. It's about shifting gears from defying time to aligning with its tempo with poise. One doesn't just stumble upon the later chapters of life unscathed; it takes thoughtful preparation to meet them head-on, the kind that dispels fear and nurtures acceptance. Consider the notion that while we invest in maintaining our zest, we must equally cultivate a resilient grace for when life's pace inevitably decelerates. To honor our lived experiences, we lean into understanding the complex harmony of emotional, physical, and legal threads that compose the tapestry of our golden years. As we explore the uncharted terrains of our own stories, we gather the threads, weaving them into a safety net for ourselves and those we hold dear, ensuring that our final acts are not mired in disarray, but instead marked by the dignified resolution of a life well-lived.

Understanding and Accepting the Later Stages of Life marks an introspective chapter that sails into the twilight years of a person's journey. Here, we delve into coming to terms with the shifts that age inevitably brings about. There's this unspoken dialogue with time that hums beneath the surface of our skin, whispering that each tick of the clock charts the course of one's life in an elaborate dance of existence and change. As the sun begins to dip lower on the horizon, acknowledging and embracing the later stages is not just an act of acceptance, but a powerful form of empowerment.

Finding tranquility in the countdown of days can be likened to an art—one that requires a serene mind and the courage to face the ephemeral nature of life. Let's unpack the baggage that comes with aging—the fears, the myths, and the unknowns—and place them under a gentle light of understanding. The narrative of our lives isn't solely written during the zealous sprints of youth but also in the measured steps of later years. Those years deserve recognition for their profound impact on the fullness of a life well-lived.

It is essential to recognize the strength in vulnerability that aging manifests. The later stages of life can lead to a natural reduction in physical vigour or agility, and this may initiate a redefining of one's self-image. How we adapt to these changes, how we retell our stories of self to ourselves, lays the groundwork for how we experience the autumn of our lives. There's an inherent beauty in celebrating the wisdom gathered rather than lamenting the fading of youth's bloom.

Lest we forget, aging is a universal chapter in life's great narrative. This shared human condition offers us an exquisite tapestry, interwoven with strands of experiences that inform and shape us. There comes a time when the days of bounding up the stairwell two steps at a time are tenderly replaced by the mindful ascent, taking each step with respectful deliberation. Embracing these adjustments is not defeat—it is an artful dance of adaptation.

As bodies evolve, so too should our living spaces. Adapting one's environment to accommodate the needs that emerge through aging is a form of self-respect, allowing one to navigate life with grace and safety. Making conscious decisions about home layouts, fixture updates, and even the tools used in daily life can make a significant difference in maintaining independence and quality of life.

Planning for the future isn't merely about saving for retirement or picking out a holiday destination. It also includes being proactive about our health—scheduling regular check-ups, staying informed about medical history, and understanding potential hereditary conditions. Partnering with healthcare providers to manage health proactively can ensure that quality care continues as one ages.

Furthermore, mental health remains an indispensable facet of aging. Cultivating strong, enduring social connections can provide a cushion against loneliness, a significant challenge during the later stages of life. By fostering a robust social network, we bolster our emotional resilience, promoting longevity and a richer, more connected life journey.

Yet, the mind, like the body, needs its own regimen of care. Engaging in activities that challenge and stimulate cognitive functions can help maintain brain health. Puzzles, games, continuous learning, and even rich conversations can serve as a workout for the mind, keeping it pliable and strong amidst the advancing years.

When we look at longevity, the spectrum extends far beyond just surviving—it's about thriving. A life well-lived isn't measured solely by the passage of years but by the joys, experiences, and wisdom those years contain. Recognizing and fostering what brings happiness and fulfillment is just as vital in the later chapters as in the opening pages of life's book.

Legal and ethical considerations too play a significant role in preparing for the years ahead. Understanding one's options regarding health directives, estate planning, and even discussing these matters with loved ones, allows for clarity and peace of mind. Such preparation ensures that an individual's wishes are respected and facilitates the transition for those who stand alongside us in our journey.

And what of the spirit? As the external pace slows, there lies a profound opportunity for inward exploration. Mindfulness and meditation can be incredible tools in nurturing a sense of peace and presence. Tapping into this spiritual wellspring can be a source of solace and wisdom, allowing one to age not just with grace but with a transcendental sense of being.

Let's remember, accepting the later stages of life doesn't mean conceding to a lower standard of existence. Far from it—it's about acknowledging the spectrum of life's stages and embracing each one with the same zest and love as the rest. It's about preparing for change, yes, but also about living out each day with joy and intention, no matter the number it holds.

It's time to shift the paradigm and see the latter years not as a quiet fade out but as a period rich with potential, growth, and continued contributions to the world. Our later years can be filled with pursuits that earlier life's demands may have prevented us from exploring fully—artistic endeavors, volunteer work, lifelong learning, or simply the cultivation of a long-neglected hobby.

Ultimately, understanding and accepting the later stages of life is an invitation to live authentically, fully, and on one's own terms. It calls for a celebration of the journey, an embrace of the here and now, and an enthusiasm for all the moments still to come. It's about respecting the past, reveling in the present, and approaching the future with a wise heart and an open mind.

As we turn the page to this vital chapter, we find ourselves entwined in the delicate balance of all that aging entails. Yet, through this guided exploration, we discover not a lament over fading youth, but a banner of honor raised high for the wisdom, experience, and beauty that only time can bestow upon us.

Legal and Ethical Considerations of Aging As we explore the panorama of strategies that pave the way for graceful aging, it's paramount to steer our conversation through the terrain of legality and moral imperatives. In this domain, the intricacies unravel—woven with threads of autonomy, rights, responsibilities, and societal constructs—that shape the dignity and quality of life as we age. Indeed, confronting the legal and ethical considerations of aging is an intricate dance—one where every step counts.

Let's first contemplate the principle of autonomy—a cornerstone of both ethical and legal frameworks. As we age, maintaining control over personal decisions is a rallying cry for dignity. Whether it's choosing where to live, consenting to medical treatments, or determining end-of-life care, the ability to self-govern is non-negotiable. However, the reality isn't always cut and dry. Cognitive decline, for instance, introduces a complex layer, challenging our capacity to make informed decisions and pushing the discussion into the realms of guardianship and power of attorney.

Now, toss into the mix the issue of consent, particularly in healthcare. Aging individuals need to be at the helms of their treatment decisions, but again, it's tricky terrain. What does informed consent truly mean for someone who may be grappling with memory loss or diminished comprehension? Legal guidelines and practice standards, while aiming to safeguard patient autonomy, also must protect the vulnerable from unwittingly making choices against their best interests.

Turning to the legal sphere, estate planning surfaces as a behemoth. It's about wills and trusts, sure, but it's also the clearest statement one can make about personal wishes for the future. And let us not underestimate the significance of advance directives—these legal documents are the crystal balls of our medical futures, offering clarity in times when we may not be able to speak for ourselves. It's a profound expression of autonomy, punctuated by the full stop of ethical principle.

However, let's not ignore the ethical quagmire presented by anti-aging interventions. Should we dive headfirst into every innovation that promises extended youth? The moral compass here swings between the drive to push boundaries and the wisdom to recognize natural processes. It's ethical curiosity walking hand in hand with prudent skepticism.

And there's the matter of access which can't be swept under the rug. In the universe of anti-aging therapies, who gets to sip from this purported fountain of youth? Ethically speaking, it's a quagmire. Equity stands tall demanding fair distribution, while practicality whispers of costs and resources. This isn't just about who can afford what, but also about who decides what's worthwhile and who benefits from the advancements in anti-aging medicine.

Privacy, in this age of digital footprints, is another plot thick with twists. Aging populations are increasingly online, navigating telemedicine and electronic health records. Herein lies a delicate balance between leveraging technology for better health outcomes and safeguarding the intimate details of one's life and body from ubiquitous data breaches.

Ageism, the lurking bias that too often seeps into the interstices of society, is a point of ethical contention. It's an insidious force that belies the value of elder wisdom and experience. Confronting ageism isn't just a battle of attitudes; it's a quest to dismantle systemic inequalities that deprive the aging population of their rightful place in society. Laws may combat blatant discrimination, but ethics demands a dismantling of the prejudices that brew beneath the surface.

Let's not sidestep the harsh reality of abuse and neglect, areas where legal and ethical lines converge with a stark warning sign. Elder maltreatment, in its many guises—be it physical, emotional, or financial—requires a vigilant society and robust legal mechanisms to defend those who may not have the strength to defend themselves.

Furthermore, the ethical dialogue on rationing healthcare is heated and heavy with implications. As resources ebb and flow, the aging populace spirals into the center of the debate. Is there a fair way to allocate limited medical resources? Ethics holds the gavel, hoping to render a verdict that honors both the collective good and the sanctity of individual lives.

Meanwhile, the legal community continues to wrestle with the ever-evolving landscape of medical aid in dying. Philosophical convictions intersect with personal beliefs, and legality binds itself to the individual's right to self-determination. Where countries and states diverge in their statutes, the ethical conversation pulses at the heart of the matter, unearthing the profound questions about life and its natural culmination.

Alignment of intergenerational family dynamics is not just the stuff of heartfelt dramas; it's an open forum for ethical debate. When parents age and roles reverse, the struggle to respect autonomy while providing necessary care often results in a tightrope walk of familial relations, fraught with potential legal tangles around caregiving decisions and shared assets.

In the same breath, it's essential to ruminate on the ethics of caregiving itself. The caregiver's burden is often heavy, threaded with duty and affection. There is an ethical mandate to support these unsung heroes who manage medications, decipher healthcare systems, and offer the comfort of companionship—yet legal and social structures are still catching up to provide the requisite scaffolding.

The dialogue would be incomplete without acknowledging the role technology plays in determining quality of life and ethical boundaries for the aged. Innovations like AI caregivers and smart homes present a cornucopia of legal and ethical questions about privacy, consent, and the very nature of human interaction.

As we unfurl the threads of the ethical and legal tapestry that colors the aging lifetime, it's clear that the interplay between the two is as complex as it is critical. Navigating these waters with a compass calibrated by empathy, respect, and justice might not make the journey easy, but it surely makes it right. To age with grace is to balance on the fulcrum of rights and responsibilities, always guided by the star of dignity.

Chapter 25:
Creating Your Personal Anti-Aging Plan

Now that we've explored the multitude of facets that play a role in longevity—from the puzzles of genetics and environmental influences on aging to proactive lifestyle choices like nutrition, exercise, and stress management—it's time you charted your own course through this complex terrain. Crafting your personal anti-aging plan isn't about hunting for a mythical fountain of youth or adhering to an impossibly rigid regimen; rather, it's about making informed, sustainable changes that fit seamlessly into your life, changes that feel less like obligations and more like second nature. With a blend of wisdom fastened from the diverse territories of science, psychology, and holistic health, assembling your plan becomes a fine balance of being realistic about where you're at and ambitious about where you want to go. By setting clear but flexible goals and checking in with your progress regularly, you'll be able to pivot as necessary, ensuring your strategy is attuned not just to the latest research, but also to the ever-changing dynamics of your own body and lifestyle. Remember, the path to a healthier, longer life is distinctly your own—no one else's blueprint will do. And while aging is an inescapable journey we all share, your map for navigating it can be as unique as your DNA.

Setting Achievable Goals Navigating the labyrinth of aging gracefully is no small feat, but with the right direction and achievable goals, it's a journey that promises rewards at every twist and turn. As we explore the nuances of creating a personal anti-aging plan in this chapter, we venture into the practical realms of setting goals that don't just sparkle in the distance but are truly within your grasp.

The first step in setting achievable goals is to dream with precision. See, it's one thing to say you want to 'stay healthy as you age,' but to actualize this nebulous desire, we must chisel it down to its finer parts. Specificity is your unwavering ally in this process. Instead of a general wish, consider what dimensions of health most resonate with your vision for aging. Is it maintaining sharp cognitive function, achieving a level of physical fitness, or fostering deeper social connections? The act of defining your goals with dead-on accuracy sets the stage for a plan that's tailored and tactical.

A sense of measurability cinches the gap between speculative and attainable goals. How nifty it is to inject your goals with metrics that allow you to track progress! Steer away from undetermined goals like 'improve strength.' Instead, aim for something quantifiable such as 'perform 20 consecutive push-ups.' Measurable goals have the knack for downing the ambiguity that so often gums up the works.

Attainability is the cornerstone of any effective goal-setting exercise. There's a delicate balance to strike here, where ambitions must be hoisted high enough to inspire yet remain sufficiently grounded to not drift into the realm of fantasy. Reflect on your current health status, resources, and time constraints. Through this lens, contemplate if your goal, though challenging perhaps, is genuinely within your reach.

Relevance weighs heavily too. The goals you etch should resonate with your personal values and larger life ambitions. If the quest for anti-aging aligns with your deep-seated values of vitality, your drive to achieve the goals will naturally amplify. Make each goal a fitting piece of the puzzle in your larger picture of well-being.

Time-bound goals exude a sense of urgency and commitment. A goal without a deadline can be eternally postponed. Whether you peg your objective to be met in three months, or a year, the ticking clock will serve as a gentle prod to keep you striding forward.

Moving beyond the SMART criteria, reflect on your whys. Understanding the substantial reasons behind each goal forges a connection that can withstand the ebb and flow of motivation. Your why could stem from a desire to play with your grandchildren without getting winded, or perhaps to embark on travels without the shadow of health concerns. In the tapestry of reasons, find those threads that hold the most meaning for you.

Prepare for setbacks, for they are inevitable. Embracing the possibility of hiccups doesn't equate to defeatism but rather primes you for resilience. When a goal seems to slip like sand through your fingers, reassess and recalibrate, don't surrender. It's all part of a dynamic process that shapes goals to be more in sync with real-world conditions.

Visualizing success is a potent tool in the goal-setting arsenal. The mind can be a fertile ground for planting the seeds of achievement through regular visualization. Imagine the outcomes, feel them as if they are present realities, and then bridge the gap with consistent action.

Accountability is another handy aide. Whether you partner with a friend, join a support group, or declare your intentions to family, being answerable to someone other than yourself raises the stakes. It can be a powerful motivator—fuel for when the initial spark dims.

Micro-goals serve as the stepping stones to grand aspirations. Want to adopt a Mediterranean diet for its longevity benefits? Start with incorporating one meal per day that fits the bill. Breaking down larger goals into digestible bites makes the journey less daunting and victories more frequent.

Transitioning from intention to habit is elemental in achieving your anti-aging goals. And habits are honed through repetition coupled with triggers and rewards. Establishing routines around your goals embeds them into the fabric of your daily life, setting the stage for long-term success.

A feedback loop is key to refining your approach. Keep a record of your progress, and schedule regular reviews. This reflective practice allows you to see what's working and what isn't and prompts adjustment. Morphing your plan based on feedback ensures it remains a living blueprint that evolves with you.

Patience is your ally in the pursuit of anti-aging goals. We often overestimate what can be achieved in the short term and underestimate the long-term possibilities. Cultivating patience wards off frustration and fosters a perspective focused on sustainable growth.

Celebrating progress, no matter how minor, fuels the drive to continue. Reward yourself for the steps taken, for they are essential components of the marathon towards aging gracefully. These celebrations are oases of joy in your quest, making the path not just fruitful but enjoyable.

In closing, setting achievable goals is less about reaching a utopian endpoint and more about crafting a journey characterized by growth, adaptation, and consistent strides toward the best version of yourself amid the tides of time. Next, we'll examine how to monitor your progress and adjust strategies, ensuring that your personalized anti-aging blueprint is not just a static document, but a dynamic approach to a vibrant life.

Monitoring Progress and Adjusting Strategies As we delve into the journey of personal transformation and embrace the strategies laid out for aging gracefully, it's vital to recognize that managing our aging process is an ongoing work in progress. Staying in tune with our bodies and minds is akin to a gardener tending to their garden, constantly observing and adjusting as the seasons change and plants grow.

Monitoring progress isn't just about watching numbers on a scale or ticking days off a calendar. It's a more nuanced, reflective process that requires us to pay attention to how we feel, both physically and mentally, as we implement the anti-aging strategies we've discussed. You'll find that tracking your energy levels, mood, cognitive functions, and physical capabilities offers insight into the effectiveness of your anti-aging regimen.

To begin with, you might consider keeping a journal. Documenting your daily experiences — the foods you eat, your exercise routines, sleep patterns, and even stress levels can reveal patterns that you otherwise might overlook. Over time, these entries become a rich database of personal health information, shedding light on what's working and what isn't.

As you pore over this information, you'll notice that certain things you're doing have a significant positive impact, while others don't seem to make much difference, or might even be counterproductive. The catch is, it's essential to give each strategy a fair chance before making judgments. In the realm of anti-aging, many practices take time before they show observable results.

Let's say you've adjusted your diet to include more anti-inflammatory foods, but after a few weeks, you're not feeling the profound changes you expected. Instead of getting discouraged, remind yourself that the internal effects, such as reduced oxidative stress or enhanced cellular repair, might not translate into immediate, visible benefits. Patience is indeed a virtue when experimenting with lifestyle changes.

Furthermore, when it comes to physical activity, tracking progress can be highly motivating. Whether you're taking up Tai Chi, hitting the gym, or simply walking more, measuring your endurance, strength, and flexibility over weeks and months will showcase your body's adaptability and resilience. But remember, it's perfectly normal for progress to ebb and flow.

If, after a considerable amount of time, certain aspects of your program aren't yielding the benefits you were aiming for, it's time to reassess. Adjusting your strategies might mean tweaking your routines — perhaps you need more sleep, a different type of exercise, or a slight change in your diet. The key is to listen to your body and be willing to adapt.

Collaborating with healthcare professionals can also provide a clearer picture of your progress. Routine medical check-ups, as recommended in previous chapters, often unveil the inner workings of our physiology that aren't immediately apparent. Blood tests, for instance, can reveal how well your body is managing oxidative stress and inflammation, two key players in the aging process.

Another aspect to consider is the role of stress and how it affects your overall well-being. Stress management techniques should lead to noticeable changes in your stress perception and resilience. If you find that your current methods aren't helping, it could be an indication that you need to explore different avenues of stress relief, such as mindfulness, which has been shown to have profound effects on psychological aging.

Technology can also serve as an incredible ally in this quest. There are a plethora of apps and devices designed to track various health metrics, from sleep quality to steps walked to calories consumed. Utilizing these tools can simplify the process of monitoring your health and provide tangible data to base your adjustments on.

Embrace the mindset that this whole process is an experiment of one — you. What works for one person might not work for another, and that's perfectly fine. Your genetic makeup, lifestyle, and personal preferences are unique, and your anti-aging strategy should be as well. Continuously learning about your body's responses and adapting your approach accordingly is the hallmark of a truly personalized anti-aging plan.

It's also important not to underestimate the power of social connections in tracking progress. Share your goals and experiences with friends, family, or even online communities. They can offer support, share their own insights, and might even help you stay accountable to your plan. Plus, social interactions themselves are a key component of a longevity-focused lifestyle, as we've discovered.

Ultimately, staying committed to monitoring and adjusting your anti-aging strategies is not just about extending your lifespan. It's about enhancing the quality of those extra years. You're ensuring that as you age, you're not just surviving, but thriving — mentally sharp, physically active, and filled with a zest for life that doesn't have to fade as the years pass.

Remember that your journey towards aging gracefully is just that — a journey. There will be bumps in the road, unexpected twists, and turns, and times when it feels like you're not making progress. That's all part of the experience. Keep your eye on the long game, and remember: small, consistent adjustments over time can lead to significant, lifelong rewards. Stay vigilant, be adaptable, and most of all, stay committed to your well-being. It's the wisest investment you can make.

Chapter 26:
The Future is Forever Young

The final pages of this journey are upon us, where we converge at the meeting point of what's known and what lies ahead in the enigmatic world of aging. We can't help but reflect on the emphatic dance of time – a siren call reminding us that while the clock ticks uniformly for all, our individual responses to its melody are varied and unique.

The past chapters have unfurled a tapestry of strategies, sciences, and stories. From the genetic threads that weave through our biological clocks to the psychological frameworks that shape our perception of aging, we've explored myriad pathways to maintaining youthfulness both within and without. Yet, as we peer into the horizon, what becomes clear is that the pursuit of longevity is not a chase for perpetual adolescence but an endeavor to thrive in every moment the universe generously lends us.

Nutritional guidance, hydration, and the very best of exercises have been handed to you like a map to a lost fountain, while sleep patterns and stress management served as the compass and sextant, navigating us through the rocky terrains of life's adversities. As we adhere to these lifestyle choices, we bolster our defenses against the siege of time, but we also come to understand that it's about the quality, not just the span, of our years that truly counts.

Skin care, once a superficial concern, has been revealed as a narrative of self-care, and hormonal health springs up as a cornerstone of vitality. The brain we've discovered is no mere organ but a garden that blooms with the right mental exercises and nutrients. Through the book, we've dispelled myths and unearthed the science-backed truths that guide us toward maintaining our cognitive vigor.

In an era where isolation threatens our well-being, social connections emerge as the elixir of life, knitting the fabric of our existence into a colorful mosaic of faces, stories, and relationships that sustain us. As humans, we're reminded that our nature is indisputably communal, and therein lies a potent antidote to the weariness of age.

And yet, while remaining rooted in age-old wisdom, we've branched into the innovations of modernity—personalized medicine, genetic testing, and the breakthroughs of anti-aging medicine, all part of our arsenal against the wiles of time. These scientific advancements extend an invitation not just to a prolonged life but to targeted, personalized approaches that consider our unique individuality.

Mindfulness and meditation, far from the mystical, have grounded themselves in the tangible realms of health and longevity, gifting us with tools to combat the stresses that seek to erode our essence. Financial health, too, weaves its way into our well-being, for a mind unburdened by economic strain is a sanctuary for youthful spirits.

The environments we choose to inhabit, the spaces we call home, are more than shelters; they are extensions of ourselves and have the profound ability to foster our wellbeing. Just as travel and adventure inject vigor into our years, our homes should serve as bastions of peace and vitality, fortifying us against the ages.

It's with this knowledge that each thread of insight intertwines—fashion and identity carving out our presence in the world, routine medical checkups safeguarding our physical form, and the lessons from longevity's elite, the celebrated Blue Zones, encouraging us to lay down a lifestyle that outpaces even the most bullish of genetics.

Yet, as we've traversed each of these avenues, we've always held the torch of consideration for the final leg of life's race. Preparing for a graceful transition, an acceptance of life's later stages, and legal ethics nestle themselves quietly yet persistently into the pages, reminding us that true preparation for aging means envisaging its full arc.

In the creation of your personal anti-aging plan, we've not sought to make claims of immortality. No, what we've hoped for is to guide you into curating a life so vivid, so rich in health and happiness, that each day feels like an ample lifetime in itself.

And now, let us pause at the threshold of this finale and turn our gaze forward, to the unchartered 'forever young' that beckons. It's a future sculpted not just by the ultimate outcomes but the daily choices—each meal, every heartbeat of exercise, and every restorative slumber. It's a future where 'young' is redefined not by years unspent but by vibrancy woven into every aspect of being.

What lies ahead is as much a discovery as it has ever been, but equipped with the knowledge you now hold, it's a discovery with a difference. You're no longer a passive traveler through time. You're now the architect of your own fountain, your personal elixir mixed from the rich well of life-augmenting wisdom garnered from every chapter, ready to drink deep from the cup of a future that's forever young.

So, take heart, for this is not an ending but a heralding of new beginnings—a continuous renewal of body, mind, and spirit, where every day is an opportunity to redefine the boundaries of our potential. As we close this book, remember that its spine does not hold the final word on your journey. You do. Let the pages of your life flourish with the youthfulness of spirit that no clock can confine nor calendar constrain. The future is, indeed, forever young.

Appendix A:
Anti-Aging Resources

Embarking on a journey to manage aging isn't just about understanding the theoretical; it's also about equipping yourself with the right tools and connections to bring those concepts to life. In this spirit, we present a curated selection of anti-aging resources designed to support you in the practical application of the strategies discussed throughout this book.

Online Platforms and Websites

National Institute on Aging (NIA): For up-to-date information on aging research and educational materials, the NIA's website is a treasure trove of scientifically vetted resources.

Mayo Clinic Healthy Aging: Renowned for reliable medical information, their section on healthy aging offers practical tips, patient care options, and healthy living strategies.

American Federation for Aging Research (AFAR): AFAR provides a wealth of insights into the latest research and findings in the field of aging.

Blue Zones: Detailed insights into the lifestyles of the world's longest-lived people, with actionable tips for incorporating their habits into your own routine.

Books and Publications

Your genes aren't always your destiny. Understanding how you can influence them is the first step to a longer life, a comprehensive guide to the genetics of aging and lifestyle interventions.

Staying Hydrated: The Secret Ingredient to Ageless Health, which unveils the myriad ways water keeps our bodies in prime condition.

Recipes for Longevity, a cookbook filled with delicious, anti-aging recipes that focus on superfoods and nutrient-rich ingredients.

Support Groups and Communities

Local and online communities play a pivotal role in maintaining motivation and sharing knowledge. Look into:

Senior Centers: Offering programs and activities that promote wellness and social connectivity for older adults.

Online Forums: Digital platforms where individuals share tips, experiences, and support each other in their anti-aging journeys.

Professional Networks

If specialized advice is what you're after, constructing a network of professionals can guide you through personalized anti-aging interventions:

Dietitians and Nutritionists who specialize in aging and longevity.

Exercise Physiologists or Personal Trainers with experience in senior fitness.

Health Coaches who provide holistic wellness and anti-aging strategies.

To maintain your edge, staying abreast of anti-aging research and development can be empowering. Attend webinars, subscribe to newsletters from top aging research institutions, and don't shy away from reaching out to experts in the field. Networking can often lead to insights and resources that are not widely known or available.

Remember, longevity isn't just about extending years to life, but also adding life to those years. With this array of resources, you'll be well-equipped to thread the pathway to a full, vibrant, and healthful future, navigating the intricacies of aging with savvy and grace.

Glossary of Terms

Navigating the landscape of longevity, we encounter numerous terms that might need clarification. Below, you'll find a curated glossary of terms to provide you with clear, concise definitions, bridging the gap between complex concepts and their practical implications in our quest for ageless vitality.

Antioxidants

Substances that inhibit oxidation, a chemical reaction that can produce free radicals, potentially leading to cell damage. Antioxidants are found in various foods and may help protect against certain diseases.

Bioavailability

The rate at which a substance is absorbed into the bloodstream and used by the body. Higher bioavailability means the body can use more of the ingested nutrient.

Cognitive Function

The mental processes that include thinking, knowing, remembering, judging, and problem-solving. These are higher-level functions of the brain, encompassing language, imagination, perception, and planning.

Detoxification

The physiological or medicinal removal of toxic substances from the human body. Detoxification aims to support and enhance the body's natural detoxification processes.

Endocrine System

A network of glands that secrete hormones into the bloodstream to regulate various bodily functions, including growth, metabolism, and sexual development.

Free Radicals

Atoms or molecules with an unpaired electron that are highly reactive and can damage cells, proteins, and DNA by altering their chemical structure. They can lead to oxidative stress.

Genetics

The study of genes, genetic variation, and heredity in living organisms. In terms of aging, genetics can determine the predisposition to certain conditions and the biological aging process.

Hydration

The process of providing an adequate amount of liquid to bodily tissues. Hydration is crucial for maintaining bodily functions and supporting overall health.

Inflammation

The immune system's response to infection or injury, which can cause redness, warmth, swelling, and pain in the affected area. Chronic inflammation is linked to various age-related diseases.

Longevity

The length or duration of a person's life. In the context of this book, it refers not just to life span but to the quality and healthfulness of those years.

Metabolism

The entirety of an organism's chemical processes. These processes are the basis of life at the molecular level, including the conversion of food into energy.

Mindfulness

A mental state of awareness, focus, and openness, which allows a person to engage fully in what they are doing at any given moment. Mindfulness is often practiced through meditation.

Nutrient Density

A measure of the amount of nutrients a food contains in comparison to the number of calories. Foods high in nutrient density provide a substantial amount of vitamins, minerals, and other beneficial substances with relatively few calories.

Oxidative Stress

A disturbance in the balance between the production of free radicals and antioxidant defenses. This condition can lead to cell and tissue damage and is a notable factor in the aging process.

Phytochemicals

Chemical compounds produced by plants. Many of these compounds are believed to be beneficial to human health and are the subject of scientific studies for their potential anti-aging effects.

Supplements

Products taken orally that contain one or more ingredients, such as vitamins, minerals, herbs, or other botanicals, intended to supplement the diet and not considered food.

This glossary isn't just an academic reference but a dynamic resource that we hope will empower you on your journey to a blissful and healthy golden era. Recall these terms as signposts guiding you through the intricate terrain of aging with grace and vigor. Let's embrace this ageless journey together, enlightened by the wisdom that each term offers to our collective quest for longevity.

www.ingramcontent.com/pod-product-compliance
Lightning Source LLC
Chambersburg PA
CBHW030319290526
45785CB00001B/435